Patient Education

Guest Editor

STEPHEN D. KRAU, PhD, RN, CNE

NURSING CLINICS OF NORTH AMERICA

www.nursing.theclinics.com

Consulting Editor
SUZANNE S. PREVOST, PhD, RN, COI

September 2011 • Volume 46 • Number 3

SAUNDERS an imprint of ELSEVIER, Inc.

W.B. SAUNDERS COMPANY

A Division of Elsevier Inc.

1600 John F. Kennedy Blvd., Suite 1800 • Philadelphia, PA 19103-2899

http://www.theclinics.com

NURSING CLINICS OF NORTH AMERICA Volume 46, Number 3
September 2011 ISSN 0029-6465, ISBN-13: 978-1-4557-1039-3

Editor: Katie Hartner
Developmental Editor: Donald Mumford

Nursing Clinics of North America (ISSN 0029-6465) is published quarterly by Elsevier Inc., 360 Park Avenue South, New York, NY 10010-1710. Months of issue are March, June, September, and December. Periodicals postage paid at New York, NY and additional mailing offices. Subscription price per year is, $135.00 (US individuals), $343.00 (US institutions), $244.00 (international individuals), $419.00 (international institutions), $197.00 (Canadian individuals), $419.00 (Canadian institutions), $74.00 (US students), and $121.00 (international students). To receive student/resident rate, orders must be accompanied by name of affiliated institution, date of term, and the signature of program/residency coordinator on institution letterhead. Orders will be billed at individual rate until proof of status is received. Foreign air speed delivery is included in all *Clinics* subscription prices. All prices are subject to change without notice. **POSTMASTER:** Send address changes to *Nursing Clinics*, Elsevier Health Sciences Division, Subscription Customer Service, 3251 Riverport Lane, Maryland Heights, MO 63043. **Customer Service: Telephone: 1-800-654-2452** (U.S. and Canada); **1-314-447-8871 (outside U.S. and Canada). Fax: 1-314-447-8029. E-mail: journalscustomerservice-usa@elsevier.com** (for print support) and **journalsonlinesupport-usa@elsevier.com** (for online support).

Nursing Clinics of North America is covered in *EMBASE/Excerpta Medica, MEDLINE/PubMed (Index Medicus), Social Sciences Citation Index, Current Contents, ASCA, Cumulative Index to Nursing, RNdex Top 100,* and Allied Health Literature and International Nursing Index (INI).

Printed and bound by CPI Group (UK) Ltd, Croydon, CR0 4YY

Transferred to Digital Print 2011

Contributors

CONSULTING EDITOR

SUZANNE S. PREVOST, PhD, RN, COI
Associate Dean, Practice and Community Engagement, University of Kentucky,
Lexington, Kentucky

GUEST EDITOR

STEPHEN D. KRAU, PhD, RN, CNE
Associate Professor, Vanderbilt University Medical Center, School of Nursing,
Nashville, Tennessee

AUTHORS

ROY BATTERHAM, MEd
Senior Research Fellow, Public Health Innovation, Population Health Strategic
Research Centre, Deakin University, Melbourne, Australia

KATHLEEN WALSH ESPER, RN, MS, CNE
Associate Professor, Madonna University, College of Nursing and Health,
Livonia, Michigan

JEFFRY GORDON, PhD
Professor of Educational Informatics, School of Nursing, Vanderbilt University,
Nashville, Tennessee

SUSAN M. HASENAU, PhD, RN, NNP, CTN-A
Professor, Madonna University, College of Nursing and Health, Livonia, Michigan

BOBBI HERRON, MS, ACNS-BC
Assistant Professor of Nursing, Department of Nursing, Purdue University
North Central, Westville, Indiana

THERESA INOTT, MSN, RN
Instructor, Vanderbilt University School of Nursing, Nashville, Tennessee

BETSY B. KENNEDY, MSN, RN
Assistant Professor, Vanderbilt University School of Nursing, Nashville, Tennessee

ANN MARIE KNOERL, MSN, RN, BC
Assistant Professor, Madonna University, College of Nursing and Health,
Livonia, Michigan

STEPHEN D. KRAU, PhD, RN, CNE
Associate Professor, Vanderbilt University Medical Center, School of Nursing,
Nashville, Tennessee

JENNI LIVINGSTON, MEd
Senior Research Fellow, Public Health Innovation, Population Health Strategic Research
Centre, Deakin University, Melbourne, Australia

MICHELLE MATTESON, RN, FNP/GNP-BC, PhD(c)
PhD Student, Sinclair School of Nursing; FNP, Department of Gastroenterology/
Hepatology; Division of Gastroenterology/Hepatology, Digestive Health Center,
University of Missouri, Columbia, Missouri

CATHY A. MAXWELL, PhD (c), RN, CCRN
Assistant Professor, Department of Nursing, Troy University, Troy, Alabama

RICHARD H. OSBORNE, PhD
Professor of Public Health; Director, Public Health Innovation, Deakin Population
Health Strategic Research Centre, School of Health and Social Development,
Deakin University, Melbourne, Australia

PAUL J. OSISEK, MEd, CAGS, MS
Associate Professor of Developmental Studies, Department of Social Science,
Purdue University North Central, Westville, Indiana

BARBARA K. REDMAN, PhD, MBE
Dean, Wayne State University, College of Nursing, Detroit, Michigan; Senior Fellow,
Center for Bioethics, University of Pennsylvania, Philadelphia, Pennsylvania

TODD M. RUPPAR, PhD, RN, GCNS-BC
Assistant Professor and JAHF-Atlantic Philanthropies Claire M. Fagin Fellow,
Sinclair School of Nursing, University of Missouri, Columbia, Missouri

CYNTHIA L. RUSSELL, PhD, RN, ACNS-BC, FAAN
Associate Professor, Sinclair School of Nursing, University of Missouri, Columbia,
Missouri

CAROLYN I. SPEROS, DNSc, APRN
Associate Professor of Nursing, University of Memphis, Loewenberg School of Nursing,
Memphis, Tennessee

WHEI MING SU, MA, RN, CCRN
Associate Professor of Nursing, Department of Nursing, Purdue University
North Central, Westville, Indiana

SHELLEY THIBEAU, MSN, RNC
Clinical Coordinator, Neonatal Intensive Care Unit, Ochsner Medical Center,
New Orleans, Louisiana

MARILYN S. TOWNSEND, PhD, RD
Cooperative Extension Nutrition Specialist, Nutrition Department, University of California
at Davis, Davis, California

Contents

> Chronic disease self-management is a growing field yet few systematic measures of its impact exist. The Health Education Impact Questionnaire (heiQ)–rigorously developed in partnership with key stakeholders–is a panel of eight highly relevant questionnaires that has been tested and applied in many settings. Wide uptake across diseases has occurred because it resonates with patient concerns, helps researchers and practitioners develop quality services, and assists policy-makers to appreciate the value of self-management support interventions. The heiQ continues to be adapted for new uses and applications creating a web of knowledge of the value and impact of health education programs.

> Medication nonadherence is a challenging and prevalent problem in older adults. Effective medication management involves successfully completing a complex group of behaviors. Meta-analyses and narrative review findings support limited benefits to medication adherence with interventions preoccupied with personal characteristics, intention, and motivation. Evidence supports a paradigm shift toward changing personal systems in which the person lives to improve and maintain medication adherence behavior. Personal-systems change systematically improves individual systems through collaboratively shaping routines, involving supportive-others in routines, and using medication self-monitoring to improve and maintain behavior. Other advances that support personal systems change are also presented.

> Patient education has long been central to nursing's philosophy of practice, and, because of this commitment, nurses in all practice settings have been deeply distressed with the careless and generally incomplete manner in which it is practiced in the health care system. This article examines the ethical underpinning of this distress and of this neglect in patient education and what actions nurses can take to correct this situation.

> Millions of Americans are living with, and managing, their chronic health
> problems. Patient education plays an essential role in promoting safe
> self-management practice. To ensure that patients attain the required abil-
> ities, patient education needs to be competency-based. When developing
> and applying a competency-based patient education lesson/program,
> each nurse must answer questions concerning essential competencies,
> optimal teaching methods, best method to evaluate patient achievement,
> and documentation of evidence. This article describes how the authors
> used these questions as a guide to achieve congruence among intended
> learning, instruction, and evaluation to design and implement a patient ed-
> ucation program, Managing Heart Failure, at a local hospital.

> Whenever the nurse encounters a patient or a patient's family, there is
> a transfer of information that is expected to be incorporated into the pa-
> tient's overall outcome. Objectives help guide the transfer of knowledge
> and provide a basis by which to evaluate the extent of the patient's under-
> standing. Bloom's Taxonomy has been a cornerstone for the development
> of objectives in academe for over half of a century. The Revised Bloom's
> Taxonomy is a tool that can be used by nurses who educate patients to
> ensure the education session is focused, clear, has standards for evalua-
> tion, and is well documented.

> Nurses must facilitate and support patient and family decision-making and
> improvement in health outcomes using instructional skills. Complex pa-
> tient needs and nursing responsibilities necessitate thoughtful consider-
> ation for maximizing the effectiveness of patient teaching encounters.
> This article reviews assessment of patient learning styles in combination
> with context for an individualized approach, as well as motivation for adult
> learners as a framework for organization of patient teaching. Methods and
> modes of patient teaching are discussed as well as tips for overcoming
> barriers to planning and implementing patient teaching.

> It is imperative that nursing responds to the call of creating a health literate
> society by taking an active role in health literacy research, education, and
> promotion. Nurses have a professional and ethical obligation to communi-
> cate in a clear, purposeful way that addresses the unique information
> needs of each patient. Evidence-based strategies that promote health lit-
> eracy must be incorporated in every patient's plan of care and become

part of the routine practice of nursing. The goal of all patient interactions should be to empower the patient to obtain, understand, and act on information that is needed for optimal health. This article explores the concept of health literacy and its relationship to patient education and communication. Practical strategies that the nurse can use to assess, communicate with, and evaluate comprehension in patients with low literacy skills are provided.

Ann Marie Knoerl, Kathleen Walsh Esper, and Susan M. Hasenau

Changes in demographics, economic, and political factors have affected health care delivery, while the patient population and the health care providers have continued to increase in diversity. Cultural sensitivity is a necessary component in development of comprehensive patient, family, or community health education plans. Consideration of the ACCESS Model can facilitate the development of successful interactions in providing culturally sensitive patient education programs.

Jeffry Gordon

Patients using the Internet are inundated with abundant information on health care that may be correct and may be incorrect. It is becoming the role of clinicians to enable patients to educate themselves by providing information about accurate and reliable Web sites, and to answer questions from literature that patients encounter. In addition, there is a myriad of technological advances to help patients and clinicians access, retrieve, and file information, and numerous communication tools to foster the patient-clinician dialog. This article provides an overview and some recommendations for clinicians to help patients better use information to achieve better outcomes.

Stephen D. Krau, Cathy A. Maxwell, and Shelley Thibeau

Patient education is a nursing responsibility that is often impromptu, spontaneous, and poorly documented. In many cases the patient's ability to perform a skill or task in the management of an illness or disease process affects the patient's outcome. A tool designed to evaluate patient performance guides the teaching process, promotes communication between the patient and nurse, and promotes communication among health care providers as it relates to patient performance. Nurses are in key positions to develop patient performance tools to ensure that the patient, or a patient's family member, can manage the health care requisites.

Marilyn S. Townsend

Providing educational materials for low-literate patients is an enormous challenge for nursing professionals given that 90 million adults in the health care setting have limited literacy skills. Through the use of a 5-step process, patient educational materials can be created to increase patient understanding of health messages and improve patient compliance.

THE CLINICS ARE NOW AVAILABLE ONLINE!

Access your subscription at:
www.theclinics.com

Preface

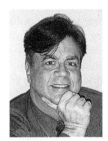

Stephen D. Krau, PhD, RN, CNE
Guest Editor

Therapeutic patient education embodies an approach to learning processes that are patient centered and focus on the needs of the patient, the resources available to the patient, the learning style of the patient, as well as the values and system of values of the patient. Effective patient education allows the patient to move from focusing on the illness or condition itself to the management and treatment of the illness, disease, risk factor, or condition. The goal of patient education focuses on the improvement of the patient's overall quality of life through objectives related to individual therapeutic compliance and preventing or reducing serious complications.

Effective patient education is the result of an integration of knowledge, skills, and motivation to modify behavior. To guide the patient, and to incorporate the patient into an educational experience, variant factors warrant consideration. This issue touches on many of the factors that are salient to an effective approach to patient education. Each article focuses on elements of those factors and provides information for the nurse to consider related to an educational approach, factors that impact the patient education, and the importance of evaluating the efficacy of the educational encounter, session, or program. These entities contribute to an evaluation process that allows the nurse to determine to what extent the educational objectives and overall goals are met to ameliorate a patient condition or illness or to prevent illness and promote health.

This issue of *Nursing Clinics of North America* provides the nurse with an overview of current thought related to the cultural aspects that impact education, ethical considerations, strategies to create objectives, as well as methods to evaluate patient ability to perform skills and tasks to meet health care demands. Research related to patient education is presented for the nurse's consideration so that creativity and individual nursing perspective can ameliorate deficits that currently exist in the arena of patient education. The importance of including the patient as a shared decision-making interaction is essential. Negotiation and patient awareness are steps that intuitively seem inherent, but without a concerted effort remain deficient. Health care providers when educating patients "only share one third of our common objectives with patients."[1]

Advances in technology have afforded nurses, patients, and other health care workers a plethora of information. As indicated by the article by Gordon, more often

doi:10.1016/j.cnur.2011.05.012

than not, it becomes the responsibility of the health care provider to help the patient decipher the information and make a determination for the best course of action for the patient. While innovative technological approaches help organize, refer, and explain patient data, it also provides opportunities for misinterpretation and confusion, which has created a new dimension for the nurse as it relates to patient education.

Evaluating the patient's learning style, and evaluating the extent to which a patient understands information or can adequately perform a skill, remains essential. Past verbal acknowledgments of patient understanding or performance abilities are limited too often to the perspective of the patient, the verbalization of the patient, with formal appraisal of what the patient has learned, or can perform. Documentation is frequently limited to acknowledgment that the patient states that they understand information, can return a demonstration, or in some cases, sign a patient education sheet. Even though the Joint Commission on the Accreditation of Health Care Organizations has set standards for patient education and documentation, actual documentation of patient education remains inadequate.[2] Signing an education sheet is evidence only that the patient has received the sheet. There is no appraisal of understanding, or even of the ability of the patient to read an educational sheet. Incorporating a more formal approach to evaluation allows the nurse to identify deficits in knowledge, skill, or motivation. A thorough health history allows an assessment of resources, learning preferences, values, and cultural variations.

Stephen D. Krau, PhD, RN, CNE
Vanderbilt University Medical Center, School of Nursing
461 21st Avenue South
Nashville, TN 37240, USA

E-mail address:
steve.krau@vanderbilt.edu

REFERENCES

1. Golay A, Lagger G, Chambouleyron M, et al. Therapeutic education of diabetic patients. Diabetes Metab Res Rev 2008;24:192–6.
2. Leisner BA, Wonch DE. How documentation outcomes guide the way: A patient health education electronic medical record experience in a large healthcare network. Qual Manag Health Care 2006;15(3):171–83.

The Evaluation of Chronic Disease Self-Management Support Across Settings: The International Experience of the Health Education Impact Questionnaire Quality Monitoring System

Richard H. Osborne, PhD*, Roy Batterham, MEd,
Jenni Livingston, MEd

KEYWORDS

- Chronic disease self management • Health education
- Questionnaire • heiQ • Evaluation

This article describes the Health Education Impact Questionnaire (heiQ).[1] its development, and main uses. It reflects on some of the knowledge revealed about the implementation of self-management support (SMS) and the quality and impact of SMS across settings in the years since its development. The heiQ is a user-friendly, relevant, and psychometrically sound instrument that provides a critical component of

The authors have nothing to disclose.
Professor Osborne was funded in part through a National Health and Medical Research Council Population Health Career Development Award. The development of the heiQ was funded in part by a research grant from the Australian Government Department of Health and Ageing.

Public Health Innovation, Deakin Population Health Strategic Research Centre, School of Health and Social Development, Deakin University, Burwood Campus, 221 Burwood Highway, Melbourne VIC 3125, Australia
* Corresponding author.
E-mail address: richard.osborne@deakin.edu.au

Nurs Clin N Am 46 (2011) 255–270
doi:10.1016/j.cnur.2011.05.010
0029-6465/11/$ – see front matter © 2011 Elsevier Inc. All rights reserved.

the comprehensive evaluation of patient education programs. The heiQ is designed be applied across a broad range of chronic conditions.

Early SMS evaluation work involved internal quality audits of an arthritis self-management program for people waiting for joint replacement surgery and a national survey through the Arthritis Foundation of Australia.[2] Although measures that were reasonable for their day were used, including a measure of self-efficacy, the data provided inadequate information to judge the effectiveness of self-management interventions and did not provide sufficiently clear information for clinicians, managers, or policymakers to improve practice. Also noted was the frustration of service providers unable to communicate the value of their SMS provision to policymakers and funders, and the frustration of policymakers who were trying to understand whether the SMS projects they had funded provided value for the money.

The heiQ was developed to address the void in the measurement of immediate and intermediate outcomes and to be used comparatively to encourage improvement in the quality of SMS delivery. SMS interventions are complex interventions[3] and, therefore, require a range of outcome indicators to support claims of effectiveness.[4–6]

To ensure that the heiQ had the greatest impact in serving the needs of all stakeholders, patients, educators, clinicians, managers, policymakers, and researchers were actively engaged in the development of the instrument. This codevelopment with key stakeholders has had a tremendous impact on the use of the instrument, as the heiQ has enjoyed rapid uptake over the past 5 years as an outcomes measure (including controlled trials), a program evaluation tool to facilitate quality monitoring and improvement (at both a local and national level), and (to a lesser extent) as a tool to enhance chronic disease care at the one-on-one patient-clinician level. Examples of the wide variety of settings, health conditions, and types of interventions where the heiQ has been used is shown in **Box 1**.

WHAT IS SMS?

The task of defining SMS is both an important step and a challenge. The field is cluttered with attempts to provide definitional clarity. For example, Bycroft and Tracey (2006)[7] cite Adams and colleagues,[8] who argue that "self management support is what health care providers, organizations and systems do to facilitate improved client self management, including provision of education and supportive interventions to increase clients' skills and confidence in managing their health problems, and includes regular assessment of progress and problems, goal setting and problem-solving support." Reference to very specific tasks in the final part of the definition has unduly limited the scope of SMS.

Although it would seem logical that the definition of SMS would be derived from a definition of self-management, historically this has not actually been the case. The Stanford approach, developed for people with arthritis by Lorig and colleagues,[9] was based on a number of key research studies in the field of health behavior change, perhaps most importantly social marketing theory and the concept of self-efficacy elucidated by Albert Bandura. Initial definitions of self-management were largely developed by Lorig's team and were related to the aims and objectives of their program. That is, self-management was what their program supported. They also developed a range of tools that further operationalized and solidified a particular understanding of both self-management and SMS. Since then there have been many attempts to broaden the concepts of both self-management and SMS, and to extend its scope to new conditions, populations, levels of complexity, and levels of need. For example, in 2005, a World Health Organization (WHO) white paper[10] described self-management as follows:

Patients will benefit from a set of cognitive and behavioral self-management skills to minimize complications or delay their onset entirely, including

- Coping skills (ie, managing emotions related to chronic conditions)
- Goal setting for specific and moderately challenging behaviors
- Self-monitoring (ie, keeping track of behaviors)
- Environmental modification (ie, creating a context to maximize success)
- Self-reward (ie, reinforcing one's behavior with immediate, personal, and desirable rewards)
- Arranging social support (ie, gaining the support of others).[10]

Our team has taken a very different approach to the matter of defining SMS and argues that, in our process of developing the heiQ, we have provided a better, grounded definition of SMS. As a starting point, we have defined the nature and scope of the ways in which patients state that they need to change to become more active participants in maintaining their health.

SMS is not a single entity and is not one-dimensional. It has evolved to include a wide range of approaches provided by health and social care services to support people with chronic and/or long-term conditions. Generally, SMS is designed to enhance patient well-being by enhancing the patient's ability to make decisions and take actions to take care of his or her health. The types of interventions to achieve these patient goals vary from therapeutically oriented one-on-one interventions to population-wide social marketing approaches.[11] At the direct face-to-face level, SMS delivery by health care professionals may involve the provision of simple written information, encouragement, or referral to more intensive care planning and support. It may also include specific skill development using motivational counseling and other techniques. Other forms of SMS include telephone coaching, Web interventions, and group programs. Population-wide approaches may use multimedia marketing approaches including television. See **Box 2** for an outline of the broad range of SMS interventions available, the intervention elements, and modes of application.

THE IMPORTANCE OF SMS

Policymakers and managers of health services, in developing and developed countries alike, are increasingly giving serious consideration to SMS for people with chronic conditions. This is because the burden of chronic disease is rapidly becoming the main contributor to loss of life and well-being, and is impinging on the effective structural and economic function of health care systems.[13–16] The number of people with chronic conditions is enormous, it is growing, and in most settings, the proportion that is being managed according to clinical guidelines is low.[17–20] This is despite numerous clinical practice guidelines explicitly including recommendations that optimum care includes patients engaging in self-management.[19,21,22] The most likely context for well-implemented SMS is where the evidence of success is irrefutable and where there is a strong and logical SMS pathway within routine care. The cardiac rehabilitation setting is a good example of this situation. Despite 48 randomized, controlled trials showing that cardiac rehabilitation reduces overall mortality by over 20% and that the intervention is cost effective, only a minority of patients receive cardiac rehabilitation.[19,20]

As with all complex and new interventions, there are many explanations for the low uptake of SMS programs across the research, clinical, and community sectors. For

Box 1
Application and uses of the heiQ

Setting
- Community health
- Disease prevention
- eHealth
- Individual treatment
- Outpatient
- Quality and Monitoring
- Screening
- Workplace rehabilitation

Users
- Charitable health care providers
- Government
- Health care professionals
- Health programs evaluators
- Hospitals
- Nongovernment organizations
- Universities

Languages
- Arabic
- Chinese
- Danish
- Dutch
- English
- French Canadian
- German
- Greek
- Italian
- Japanese
- Korean
- Macedonian
- Norwegian
- Polish
- Samoan
- Spanish
- Thai
- Tongan
- Turkish
- Vietnamese

Health conditions
- Back pain
- Cancer
- Chronic obstructive pulmonary disease
- Depression
- Diabetes
- Elderly
- Epilepsy
- Fibromyalgia
- Hemophilia
- Heart disease
- Hepatitis
- HIV
- Hyperlipidemia
- Hypertension
- Lupus
- Lymphedema
- Multiple sclerosis
- Obesity
- Osteoarthritis
- Osteoporosis
- Pain syndromes
- Parkinson disease
- Psoriasis
- Rheumatoid arthritis
- Schizophrenia
- Sight impaired
- Stroke

Intervention
- Arthritis self-management
- Back Education Course
- Bounce Back with Babies
- Breath of Fresh Air
- Cardiac rehabilitation
- Cardiopulmonary rehabilitation
- Chronic disease self-management
- Coaching
- Controlling Depression

Diabetes complications	Moving On after Stroke
Expert Patients Program	Moving Towards Wellness
Flinders Program	Multiple sclerosis—lifestyle self-help
Group strength-training	No Falls Program
Healthy Bodies	Osteoporosis self-management
Healthy Eating and Lifestyle Program	Parkinson disease self-management
Heart failure	Parkinson early management
Heartwise	Physical exercise
Hospital readmission prevention	Preparation for surgery
Impaired glucose tolerance program	Pulmonary rehabilitation
Introduction of new technology	Self-control and management of pain
Life and living residential (cancer)	Stanford Self-Management
Living Well with Diabetes	Tai Chi
Living with Rheumatoid Arthritis	Weight loss

Box 2
Key elements of SMS interventions

Key elements of interventions

Patient-centered care

Rapport, empowerment, confidence building

Coaching

Motivational counseling

Goal setting

Pacing

Tailoring to consumers needs

Modes of application of SMS

Direct contact

One-on-one

Small-group consultation

Lay-led and/or professional-led group course

Indirect contact

Written information

Web

Telephone

Text message

Mass media

Blended learning approaches[12]

Various combinations of the above modes

example, for a controlled clinical trial of the impact of group-based SMS,[23] observations of over 1000 people with hip or knee osteoarthritis showed that they are generally unwilling to attend a 6 week group program for several pragmatic reasons. They cannot travel, they are unable to sit in 2.5-hour sessions, they work during the day when courses are provided, or they do not like the group settings (Osborne RH, unpublished data, 2009). There is a perennial challenge in the provision of SMS in both the community and routine clinical setting to recruit a critical mass of patients to be able to operate group-based programs. Although much of this relates to limited availability of programs at convenient times and settings, there are also limited "entry points" or ways patients can find or be referred to ongoing SMS opportunities.

The development of solutions to the inadequate management of chronic disease is not simply a matter of directing more funding to chronic disease management but, instead, a matter of developing a whole-systems approach.[16] A whole-systems approach becomes problematic when there is limited funding, inadequate facilities, and when the health professionals usually approached to implement SMS (ie, doctors, nurses, allied health professionals) are already in short supply. Other key barriers are the lack of endorsement and referral from primary physicians, and overcrowding and lack of time in developed and developing country settings.[13,24]

THE IMPORTANCE OF CONTINUING EVALUATION OF SMS

There is growing evidence of the value of SMS through a well funded and scientific research agenda, including randomized, controlled trials.[25–29] These trials include efficacy studies, where the impact of SMS is tested under ideal conditions, and effectiveness studies, where there is an attempt to test SMS in more "real-world" circumstances.

The authors have often been asked if it is necessary to continue evaluating SMS programs when there have been many controlled trials demonstrating SMS effectiveness. Additionally, authoritative organizations have endorsed and embedded SMS into their routine work. For example, SMS programs have been endorsed by various nongovernment organizations in many countries. In the United Kingdom, it has become part of National Health Service reform. In public settings we also hear weaker arguments against ongoing evaluation based on the claims that "Patients tell us that it's working so we don't need to bother with evaluation." Although these arguments may suggest that further research is not required, the need for evaluation, particularly at the local level, is ongoing.

There are strong arguments for providers of SMS programs and services to continue to evaluate these services. First, whereas efficacy and effectiveness trials are seen as necessary, they are not always helpful for local providers and national funders, most often because they ignore the very significant role of the skilled professional provider of SMS.

Second, local providers and national funders need information from the ongoing evaluation of SMS programs. Managers and funders believe that evaluation of SMS is undertaken to demonstrate impact, to provide accountability, and to guide future decision making, including decisions about sustainability and integration. Less recognized roles include the provision of information to help improve programs at the local level and quality improvement at the national level.

Third, there is limited high quality evidence in many settings and for many models of SMS. For example, we have found that few health care providers confidently and routinely refer patients to SMS. Healthcare professionals and funders require stronger and clearer information about what works for whom in what context.

CHALLENGES IN SMS EVALUATION AND OUTCOMES ASSESSMENT

One challenging part of any research or evaluation effort is outcomes assessment. When a limited range of evaluation tools and approaches predominate, there is a risk of the scope of an intervention becoming defined and therefore constrained by the available evaluation tools. If there is a dominant approach to evaluation, such as a widely used questionnaire, that field may become defined by the specific constructs embodied in the questionnaire. When we first entered the field in the early 2000s, we were asked to evaluate the impact of SMS on people with arthritis.[2] At the same time, reviews began to suggest that SMS interventions for people with arthritis were not effective[30] although they were effective in other selected chronic conditions (eg, diabetes, asthma, and hypertension). This generated concern, as the operation of arthritis programs was a core research area and these programs were beginning to be widely endorsed.[31]

We began to examine reasons why self management interventions appear to be ineffective for people with arthritis while being effective for other diseases. Possible explanations included (1) that the intervention was ineffective and (2) that meta-analysis using a single outcome measure was not an appropriate procedure for judging the effectiveness of SMS because SMS is a complex intervention.[3] Although there was sound and wide-ranging evidence that the interventions were working, the meta-analyses undertaken by Warsi and colleagues[30] found pain and disability were the primary outcomes for self-management interventions in people with arthritis. Pain and disability were used because there is no reliable clinical indicator of arthritis outcomes. In the context of the goals of SMS, a potential reduction of pain and disability provides only a limited perspective of the potential benefits that a person with arthritis might receive. SMS programs showed that participants could improve their coping with chronic disease and participation in life despite persistent pain linked to their chronic arthritis. SMS for those with diabetes and hypertension has been associated with very clear clinical endpoints where blood levels of hemoglobin A1c or blood pressure are expected to reduce because there is a direct causal link between patient behaviors, medical interventions, and these outcomes. By contrast, in arthritis there are only subjective measures of pain and disability available. As articulated in the above citation from WHO,[10] SMS programs have a broad range of outcomes, including assisting people to adjust, cope, develop specific competencies, and have a positive life despite their ongoing chronic condition. These observations led us to consider general measures of the intended outcomes of SMS interventions rather than specific measures.

DEVELOPMENT AND APPLICATION OF THE HEIQ

The development and characteristics of the heiQ have been well described elsewhere.[1,32,33] Briefly, the principal motivation for developing the heiQ was to enable more direct and realistic measurement of the impact and quality of SMS to inform health professional and lay leaders, health practitioners, policymakers, and researchers in their work. Given that previous measures did not seem to adequately cover the full range of potential benefits, we set out to take both a patient-centered and system-centered approach, and employed grounded methods in the development of the heiQ.

In-depth consultation and program logic modeling were used to derive from clients and professionals what might be the individual and theoretical domains of outcomes. Importantly, the words that clients offered during the consultations were retained in the wording of each item in the questionnaire. The constructs that arose are presented in **Box 3**. Given the grounded process by which constructs and items were derived, the questionnaire has high content and face validity. Strong evidence of construct validity was established using a rigorous confirmatory factor analysis.[1]

It is important to note that a questionnaire can never be fully validated; rather a questionnaire acquires a web of evidence indicating its properties and utility across settings and over time.[34,35] The heiQ scales have been used by a wide variety of organizations, across settings, and in interventions for people with a very wide range of health conditions (see **Box 1**). It is has been used for quality and monitoring at the organizational, regional, or national level (eg, Australia, Canada, England, Germany, Japan, New Zealand, Thailand) and in randomized, controlled trials, some of which have published protocols or outcomes.[23,36–40]

The heiQ scales have been translated and culturally adapted into about 20 languages. An important challenge of translation is the recreation of the idiomatic expressions (common phrases or sayings whose meanings cannot be understood by the individual words or elements) that commonly arise when questionnaire items are faithfully derived from patients' own words. An example is, "My health problems do not ruin my life." If the "ruin my life" element was translated literally the intent of the item would be lost. It is reasonably well known across English-speaking cultures that this item is referring to how the condition might make life very difficult and more challenging than anticipated. To improve the fidelity of the translation and cultural adaptation, a formal protocol is followed where forward translators (translation from English to target language) are provided with an "item intent document." Following forward translation, independent translators then do back translation to English language, and then extensive consultations take place between the developer Richard Osborne, translators, and clinical and community staff who are familiar with the types of words and language sophistication used by the "average" consumer.

Additional Specific Uses and Adaptations of the HeiQ

A number of specific adaptations and applications have also taken place and some are listed below.

Cancer

Empowerment is a multifaceted concept and a challenge to measure in any context. In Canada, Maunsell and colleagues[41] tested the five heiQ scales most relevant to the empowerment construct in the cancer context: emotional well-being to distress, constructive attitudes and approaches, skill and technique acquisition (two items modified), social integration and support, and health services navigation (one item modified). In a large psychometric study, the properties of the modified heiQ were excellent, suggesting that these scales are reliable and valid measures in the psycho-oncology setting. In the United Kingdom, the heiQ is being used as an indicator of quality of cancer survival.

Workplace health promotion

In Japan, Arakida and colleagues adapted the heiQ for the evaluation of workplace health education programs designed to reduce metabolic syndrome (including being overweight, physical inactivity, and hypertension) and prevent diabetes onset. In Australia, the heiQ is being used as a secondary outcome measure in a trial of vocational rehabilitation combined with group-based SMS.[38]

Evaluation of the introduction of new technology

In the United Kingdom, the heiQ is being used alongside other measures in the Whole System Demonstrator Project led by Newman and colleagues. This is a large

Box 3
heiQ domains, keywords, and descriptors

1. Health-directed activity

   a. *Keywords: healthful behaviors, walking, exercise, relaxation*

   b. This construct relates to the level of functional activity incorporated into lifestyle. The activities may be aimed at either disease prevention and/or health promotion. Many people with chronic conditions do very little or no exercises and this scale is designed to detect small but tangible improvements.

2. Positive and active engagement in life

   a. *Keywords: engaged in life, positive affect*

   b. This construct covers motivation to be active and embodies the notion of participants in self-programs engaging or re-engaging in life-fulfilling activities because of program involvement. It includes both behavioral elements (participation in life activities) and psychological elements (enthusiasm for life activities).

3. Emotional distress

   a. *Keywords: health-related negative affect; anxiety, stress, anger, depression*

   b. This construct measures negative affective responses to illness, including anxiety, anger, and depression (which are attributed to health). The items in this construct are reversed.

4. Self-monitoring and insight

   a. *Keywords: self monitoring, setting reasonable targets, insight into living with a health problem*

   b. This construct captures how an individual engages in self-monitoring of their condition. An important component of this construct is the individuals' acknowledgment of realistic disease-related limitations, and the ability and confidence to adhere to these limits. This may also relate to the monitoring of specific subclinical indicators of disease status.

5. Constructive attitudes and approaches

   a. *Keywords: positive attitude, sense of control, empowerment*

   b. This construct is embodied in the statement "I am not going to let this disease control my life" and includes a shift in how individuals' view the impact of their condition on their life.

6. Skill and technique acquisition

   a. *Keywords: symptom relief skills, skills and techniques to manage own health*

   b. This construct aims to capture change in the knowledge-based skills and techniques (including the use of equipment) that participants acquire or relearn to help them manage with disease-related symptoms and health problems.

7. Social integration and support

   a. *Keywords: feelings of social isolation because of the illness, sense of support, seeking support from others*

   b. This construct aims to capture the positive impact of social engagement and support that evolves through interactions with others. It also involves the confidence to seek support from interpersonal relationships as well as from community-based organizations.

8. Health service navigation

   a. *Keywords: communication, decision processes, relationships with health professionals*

   b. This construct is concerned with an individual's understanding of and ability to confidently interact with a range of health organizations and health professionals. Further, it measures the confidence and ability to communicate and negotiate with health care providers to get needs met.

randomized, controlled trial of tele-care and tele-health for people with long-term conditions and those with social care needs.

National quality and monitoring
Several authorities have established systematic quality monitoring of widely applied SMS interventions. The most prominent is the Expert Patients Program in the United Kingdom (www.expertpatients.co.uk), which has incorporated the heiQ into a national Web-based system that collects and analyses heiQ data to inform course leaders and, thus, support quality of course delivery.

DEVELOPMENTS NEEDED IN RELATION TO THE HEIQ AND ITS APPLICATIONS

The heiQ was developed as a tool for evaluation and the great majority of uses described previously were clearly for evaluation of either programs conducted by specific agencies or broader regional or national programs. This section describes a number of identified issues with the heiQ and, where applicable, describes preliminary work that has been undertaken to address these needs. Generally, these issues relate to extending the use of the heiQ beyond evaluative uses and beyond chronic conditions. In summary, the issues relate to

1. The use of the heiQ for needs assessment and care planning with groups or individuals
2. Use for primary (and some secondary) prevention and for understanding well-being activities
3. Developing guidelines on when to use particular scales and how to interpret patterns of scale scores.

Use for Needs Assessment and Care Planning

One of the main difficulties with administering the tool at the individual level is that it needs to be administered by health professionals who are often reluctant to take up the time of the client in completing a tool that is not of immediate use to either of them. This is probably compounded by a feeling that the heiQ could be useful but they are not sure how to fully use the information. There have been questions as to what extent the tool can be used to give information about the needs of clients of a service (or of a group of people) at either an individual or an aggregated level. The need to develop approaches and a body of data to support these types of applications is recognized and being addressed.

There are two difficulties in using the heiQ for individual care-planning. The complexity of the scoring algorithm makes it difficult for a clinician to score the tool with immediacy. Additionally, scale scores are less likely to be reliable at the individual level than they are at the group level. In seeking to address the first issue, one of the authors has developed paper-based and computerized scoring tools that will allow a practitioner to score the eight scales in less than 3 minutes. In seeking to address the second issue, there is now a tool that enables a health practitioner to present and discuss the results with the client in a way that facilitates a clinical discussion and which gives the client an opportunity to validate his or her results. Clients and health practitioners can engage in therapeutic conversations as a result of examining heiQ scales because the items given contain the intent and wording that were derived directly from clients during the tool's development.

There are two options for using the tool to understand and plan for the needs of groups. Both of these options involve considering the results as a profile of scores across the eight scales. The first approach focuses on the average score on each scale and compares this with national or international averages. This helps to determine to what extent a particular group may have higher or lower needs in any of the measured areas than the norm.

The second approach focuses on understanding the variation within the target group by looking at the different patterns of scores across the eight heiQ scales. For example, it is known that there is a pattern that is quite common in people who are newly diagnosed with their condition. Typically, they score very high on emotional distress, health-related activity, and self-monitoring and insight. It could be said that this group of people is anxious and hypervigilant. It would be a mistake to offer these people SMS interventions that make them feel more anxious and pressured because their main need is for assistance in putting their illnesses into some sort of manageable context in their lives. On the other hand, there is a pattern that is common in people who are older and who have lived with an illness for some years. Typically these people score low on emotional distress but also low on positive and active engagement in life and low on self-monitoring and insight. Many of these people have adapted to a lower set of expectations about their life, and a key SMS strategy may be to link them into activities and social networks that help them regain enthusiasm for life.

Both of these options for using the heiQ to identify and understand the needs of groups require reliable benchmarking data across nations, people in particular age groups and with particular conditions, as well as descriptors of common profiles. There is also a need for research into effective SMS strategies for groups with different patterns of need. There is currently a collaborative effort in process to create benchmarking and profile descriptors as well as intervention options. National benchmarks are already well established in Australia. In the United Kingdom, derived benchmarks will soon be available.

Applicability to Primary Prevention

It is recognized that the heiQ was developed in the context of evaluation of chronic disease programs; many of the scales are relevant to prevention programs as well as to health and well-being–related behaviors in the general population. Indeed, some of the scales require adaptation to suit the situation of secondary prevention in individuals who have asymptomatic diseases. This is well advanced in Japanese workplace health-promotion settings and for cancer empowerment. In these settings, the psychometric structure needs to be reconfirmed in relevant target populations and such studies are near completion.

Guidelines for Use and Reporting Particular heiQ Scales

The question is often asked as to whether the heiQ is suitable for the evaluation of a particular intervention. The answer is always the same: "It depends!" It is crucial that clinicians, researchers, policymakers, program managers, and providers carefully document the content and the intended impact of the SMS intervention they seek to evaluate. With this information, a careful match can then be made between what the intervention is intending to achieve and what evaluation tools are best suited for providing evidence with that intent in mind. It is important to note that the heiQ consists of eight separate independent questionnaires specifically designed and validated to be administered either singly or as a panel of indicators.

The heiQ items are scored on a Likert-type scale from 1 to 4, corresponding to strongly disagree to strongly agree. Each of the scales has between four and six questions. To facilitate a consistent understanding of scores, the scale score is the average of the item scores. This means the scale score can be represented on the same Likert-type scale as the individual items. Currently, there are guidelines be developed that will guide the user to calculate the proportion of SMS attendees who have the potential for a measurable change after taking part in an intervention. Updated guidelines for calculating the proportion of people who have benefited have also been created. These calculations rely heavily on sound national databases to define norms for each scale.

One of the key reasons the heiQ has had high uptake in the field is because practitioners and managers get prompt and easily understandable information about the impact and quality of the interventions they are providing as compared with a norm score. Some organizations have used a Web-based data-gathering and reporting system to facilitate cost-effective data entry, analysis, and prompt reporting. The reports provide baseline (at entry into the SMS intervention) heiQ scores showing the efficacy of targeted recruitment into the SMS intervention. When the average entry score is high, an excess of individuals will have modest or no potential to derive benefit from the intervention. There has been an attempt to estimate the magnitude of a substantial improvement that provides information about the proportion who benefit. This suggests that, for a given domain, the proportion who benefit in a high-quality intervention ranges from about 20% to greater than 60%—very much depending on entry scores, the type of disease, and the aims, quality, and intensity of the intervention. Several organizations are systematically collecting heiQ quality and impact data. These data are being used for quality improvement feedback to educators as well as to trainers, persons in management roles, and to funders.

CONTEXT FOR ADVANCEMENT OF SELFMANAGEMENT SUPPORT

The heiQ was developed in response to an obvious void in available measurement tools. Its development included the participation of not only patients, but also health care professionals, managers, and policymakers. There has been wide use of the heiQ because, during its development, there careful consideration was given to what potential users identified as their need, and because use of the tool provides the data to address the needs of their clients. There was not a guiding theory as to what the dimensions of SMS should be. The developers used a grounded approach. That is, the dimensions of SMS were discovered through genuine consumer consultation using a patient-focused process of questionnaire design that included concept mapping. Therefore, the definition of SMS that emerged is the activities that people undertake in the eight areas defined by the heiQ as presented in **Box 3**.

Since the early 2000s, the team has had the opportunity to either evaluate or to observe the evaluation of a very large range of SMS interventions. More recently, the team has had the opportunity to develop SMS and other types of interventions de novo for orthopedic waiting list reform, workplace health education, hepatitis C SMS, equitable provision of SMS in rural Thailand, and a Web-based SMS program for people with musculoskeletal disorders and mental health concerns. This experience has led to a range of insights regarding the relative success and failure of programs, as well as potential benefits and deleterious effects.

THE NEW SMS

The heiQ was developed at a time when SMS was generally thought of in terms of particular programs, both group programs and programs that involved individual goal setting and coaching. Whereas the value of these programs continues to be recognized, there has been increasing concern that these programs do not suit everyone. A major concern is that the very people who are at highest risk of serious decline in their health (and of incurring high medical and hospital costs) are, in many cases, unlikely to participate in these programs. There has been a concern that SMS may appeal primarily to people of certain educational and income levels and may result in exacerbating health inequalities. This has led to numerous calls to change the way SMS is considered. It is important that SMS be not just targeted toward those with high capacity to meet an ideal of self-management that focuses on (1) self-initiation of health care actions and access to health services, and (2) a set of particular health behavior targets.[34,42,43] People of all levels of ability and in a wide range of complex circumstances have the ability to improve their level of participation in health-related decisions and actions in ways that bring about significant heath benefits. For these reasons and others, there are increasing calls for SMS to be integrated into all service provision by agencies, especially in primary care, community health, and ambulatory care.[35,44]

New ways of thinking about and conducting SMS will require new ways of measuring the success of these endeavors. This warrants consideration for use of the heiQ in new and more systemic ways. One possibility is the incorporation of the heiQ (or relevant scales) into standard assessment and care-planning tools; this will require further development of the processes for use in individual care provision as previously discussed. A second possibility is the use of the heiQ with samples of a service's clients. This would require the development of guidelines for sampling based on the diversity of the agencies clients.

SUMMARY

SMS is a very dynamic field with rapid changes occurring in theory and practice. The heiQ was developed to meet certain evaluation needs that were identified in the early 2000s. It is a tool that will maintain its relevance through the various transitions and developments that occur in SMS but, to ensure this, we will need to maintain the same level of partnership with stakeholders as was achieved in the initial development of the tool.

ACKNOWLEDGMENTS

The authors with to thank Gerald Elsworth, Mikako Arakida, Stanton Newman, Elizabeth Mausell, Jim Phillips, Kathryn Whitfield, Crystal McPhee, Amanda Springer, Melanie Hawkins, Ian Wicks, Michael Fisher, and Graeme Rossiter. The authors also wish to acknowledge the generosity of evaluation clients who have spent time discussing the heiQ and its meaning for their programs and provided us with many valuable insights.

REFERENCES

1. Osborne RH, Elsworth GR, Whitfield K. The Health Education Impact Questionnaire (heiQ): an outcomes and evaluation measure for patient education and self-management interventions for people with chronic conditions. Patient Educ Couns 2007;66(2):192–201.
2. Osborne RH, Wilson T, Lorig KR, et al. Does self-management lead to sustainable health benefits in people with arthritis? A 2-year transition study of 452 Australians. J Rheumatol 2007;34(5):1112–7.

3. Craig P, Dieppe P, Macintyre S, et al. Developing and evaluating complex interventions: the new Medical Research Council guidance. BMJ 2008;337:a1655.
4. Lewin S, Glenton C, Oxman AD. Use of qualitative methods alongside randomised controlled trials of complex healthcare interventions: methodological study. BMJ 2009;339:b3496.
5. Shepperd S, Lewin S, Straus S, et al. Can we systematically review studies that evaluate complex interventions? PLoS Med 2009;6(8):e1000086.
6. Emsley R, Dunn G, White IR. Mediation and moderation of treatment effects in randomised controlled trials of complex interventions. Stat Methods Med Res 2010;19(3):237–70.
7. Bycroft J, Tracey J. Self-management support: a win-win solution for the 21st century. New Zeal Fam Physician 2006;33(4):243.
8. Adams K, Greiner A, Corrigan J. The first annual crossing the quality chasm summit: a focus on communities. Washington, DC: Institute of Medicine; 2004.
9. Lorig K, Gonzalez VM, Laurent DD, et al. Arthritis self-management program variations: three studies. Arthritis Care Res 1998;11(6):448–54.
10. World Health Organization. Preparing a health care workforce for the 21st century: the challenge of chronic conditions. Geneva (Switzerland): World Health Organization; 2005.
11. Jordan JE, Osborne RH. Chronic disease self-management education programs: challenges ahead. Med J Aust 2007;186(2):84–7.
12. Brinkerhoff R, Apking A. Does the E-world change everything? In: High impact learning. Cambridge (MA): Perseus Publishing; 2001. Chapter 2.
13. Wanitkun N, Batterham R, Vichathai C, et al. Building equity in chronic disease management in Thailand: a whole of system approach to introducing pro-active chronic illness care. Chronic Illn 2011;7(1):31–44.
14. Kreindler SA. Lifting the burden of chronic disease: what has worked? What hasn't? What's next? Healthc Q 2009;12(2):30–40.
15. Bodenheimer T, Chen E, Bennett HD. Confronting the growing burden of chronic disease: can the U.S. health care workforce do the job? Health Aff (Millwood) 2009;28(1):64–74.
16. World Health Organization. Innovative care for chronic conditions: building blocks for action: global report. Geneva: World Health Organization; 2002.
17. Jenssen TG, Tonstad S, Claudi T, et al. The gap between guidelines and practice in the treatment of type 2 diabetes A nationwide survey in Norway. Diabetes Res Clin Pract 2008;80(2):314–20.
18. Protheroe J, Rogers A, Kennedy AP, et al. Promoting patient engagement with self-management support information: a qualitative meta-synthesis of processes influencing uptake. Implement Sci 2008;3:44.
19. Bethell HJ, Lewin RJ, Dalal HM. Cardiac rehabilitation: it works so why isn't it done? Br J Gen Pract 2008;58(555):677–9.
20. Griffiths C, Motlib J, Azad A, et al. Randomised controlled trial of a lay-led self-management programme for Bangladeshi patients with chronic disease. Br J Gen Pract 2005;55(520):831–7.
21. Zhang W, Moskowitz RW, Nuki G, et al. OARSI recommendations for the management of hip and knee osteoarthritis, Part II: OARSI evidence-based, expert consensus guidelines. Osteoarthritis Cartilage 2008;16(2):137–62.
22. National Institute for Health and Clinical Excellence. Clinical guideline 87. Type 2 diabetes: the management of type 2 diabetes. England: NICE; 2009.
23. Osborne RH, Buchbinder R, Ackerman IN. Can a disease-specific education program augment self-management skills and improve health-related quality of

life in people with hip or knee osteoarthritis? BMC Musculoskelet Disord 2006;7: 90.

24. Rogers A, Bury M, Kennedy A. Rationality, rhetoric, and religiosity in health care: the case of England's Expert Patients Programme. Int J Health Serv 2009;39(4): 725–47.

25. Chodosh J, Morton SC, Mojica W, et al. Meta-analysis: chronic disease self-management programs for older adults. Ann Intern Med 2005;143(6):427–38.

26. Cochran J, Conn VS. Meta-analysis of quality of life outcomes following diabetes self-management training. Diabetes Educ 2008;34(5):815–23.

27. Guevara JP. Self-management education of children with asthma: a meta-analysis. LDI Issue Brief 2003;9(3):1–4.

28. Warsi A, LaValley MP, Wang PS, et al. Arthritis self-management education programs: a meta-analysis of the effect on pain and disability. Arthritis Rheum 2003;48(8):2207–13.

29. Newman S, Steed L, Mulligan K. Self-management interventions for chronic illness. Lancet 2004;364(9444):1523–37.

30. Warsi A, Wang PS, LaValley MP, et al. Self-management education programs in chronic disease: a systematic review and methodological critique of the literature. Arch Intern Med 2004;164(15):1641–9.

31. Rogers A, Kennedy A, Bower P, et al. The United Kingdom Expert Patients Programme: results and implications from a national evaluation. Med J Aust 2008; 189(Suppl 10):S21–4.

32. Nolte S, Elsworth GR, Sinclair AJ, et al. The extent and breadth of benefits from participating in chronic disease self-management courses: a national patient-reported outcomes survey. Patient Educ Couns 2007;65(3):351–60.

33. Nolte S, Elsworth GR, Sinclair AJ, et al. Tests of measurement invariance failed to support the application of the "then-test". J Clin Epidemiol 2009;62(11): 1173–80.

34. Kendall E, Ehrlich C, Sunderland N, et al. Self-managing versus self-management: reinvigorating the socio-political dimensions of self-management. Chronic Illn 2011;7(1):87–98.

35. Williams A, Dennis S, Harris M. How effective are the linkages between self-management programmes and primary care providers, especially for disadvantaged patients? Chronic Illn 2011;7(1):20–30.

36. Francis KL, Matthews BL, Van Mechelen W, et al. Effectiveness of a community-based osteoporosis education and self-management course: a wait list controlled trial. Osteoporos Int 2009;20(9):1563–70.

37. Cadilhac DA, Kilkenny MF, Lindley RI, et al. A Phase II multi-centered, single-blind, randomized, controlled trial of the Stroke Self-Management Program. Stroke 2011;42(6):1673–9.

38. Ellis N, Johnston V, Gargett S, et al. Does self-management for return to work increase the effectiveness of vocational rehabilitation for chronic compensated musculoskeletal disorders? Protocol for a randomised controlled trial. BMC Musculoskelet Disord 2010;11:115.

39. Stone GR, Packer TL. Evaluation of a rural chronic disease self-management program. Rural Remote Health 2010;10(1):1203.

40. Crotty M, Prendergast J, Battersby MW, et al. Self-management and peer support among people with arthritis on a hospital joint replacement waiting list: a randomised controlled trial. Osteoarthritis Cartilage 2009;17(11):1428–33.

41. Maunsell E, Lauzier S, Brunet J, et al. Measurement of five dimensions of patient empowerment in oncology: validation of the Health Education Impact

Questionnaire (heiQ). Melbourne (Australia): Clinical Oncological Society of Australia (COSA); 2010.

42. Vassilev I, Rogers A, Sanders C, et al. Social networks, social capital and chronic illness self-management: a realist review. Chronic Illn 2011;7(1):60–86.

43. Osborne RH, Jordan JE, Rogers A. A critical look at the role of self-management for people with arthritis and other chronic diseases. Nat Clin Pract Rheumatol 2008;4(5):224–5.

44. Jordan JE, Briggs AM, Brand CA, et al. Enhancing patient engagement in chronic disease self-management support initiatives in Australia: the need for an integrated approach. Med J Aust 2008;189(Suppl 10):S9–13.

Improving Medication Adherence: Moving from Intention and Motivation to a Personal Systems Approach

Cynthia L. Russell, PhD, RN, ACNS-BC[a],*,
Todd M. Ruppar, PhD, RN, GCNS-BC[b],
Michelle Matteson, RN, FNP/GNP-BC, PhD(c)[c,d,e]

KEYWORDS

- Medication adherence • Interventions • Patient education
- Older adults

The older population has grown tremendously, and this trend is expected to continue. At present, there are nearly 40 million adults who are 65 years and older in the United States, and this number is anticipated to double by the year 2020.[1] Chronic diseases, such as heart disease, diabetes, and stroke, are more prevalent in older adults.[2] Concomitant with these chronic diseases is the need to take a plethora of medications prescribed to treat varied disorders. An average of 8.8 medications per day is taken by older persons living at home. These medications are frequently associated with complex dosing and scheduling requirements. Although most agree that taking medications is an important strategy for managing chronic illnesses, it is estimated that about 50% of patients do not take their medications as prescribed.[3]

Effective medication management involves a complex group of behaviors, including obtaining medications from a pharmacy, administering the correct drug and dose at

The authors have nothing to disclose.
[a] S423 University of Missouri, Sinclair School of Nursing, University of Missouri, Columbia, MO 65211, USA
[b] S324 MU Sinclair School of Nursing, University of Missouri, Columbia, MO 65211, USA
[c] Sinclair School of Nursing, University of Missouri, Columbia, MO 65211, USA
[d] Department of Gastroenterology/Hepatology, University of Missouri, Columbia, MO 65203, USA
[e] Division of Gastroenterology/Hepatology, Digestive Health Center, 101 South Fairview, University of Missouri, Columbia, MO 65203, USA
* Corresponding author.
E-mail address: RussellC@missouri.edu

Nurs Clin N Am 46 (2011) 271–281
doi:10.1016/j.cnur.2011.05.004
0029-6465/11/$ – see front matter © 2011 Elsevier Inc. All rights reserved.

nursing.theclinics.com

the correct time as prescribed, and monitoring for intended and unintended effects.[2] Adherence to the prescribed medication prescription is important for achieving therapeutic drug effects. Adherence, as defined by the World Health Organization, is "the extent to which a person's behavior (taking medications, following a recommended diet and/or executing lifestyle changes) corresponds with the agreed recommendations of a health care provider."[4(p13)] Medication adherence barriers for older adults include cognitive problems; beliefs that are not congruent with medication taking; diminished hearing, sight, and touch; strained financial resources; sensitivity to medication side effects; and being prescribed a large number of medications.[5] Rates of medication nonadherence in older adults have been documented from 25% to 59% depending on population and settings.[5] More than 10% of hospital admissions for older adults may be attributed to medication nonadherence, resulting in great financial costs.[5] In the general population, financial costs of medication nonadherence have been estimated to be $300 billion.[6] In addition, medication nonadherence in older adults has been shown to result in poor quality of life and undesirable clinical outcomes.[6–9]

The purpose of this article is to review the theories and interventions that have been used in an attempt to improve medication adherence behavior in older adults. We then propose a paradigm shift, a novel medication adherence intervention that focuses on tapping into the personal system in which the individual functions to change medication-taking behavior. We discuss early successes using this innovative approach and also the future trends in research and practice with medication adherence in older adults and its practice.

MEDICATION ADHERENCE THEORIES

For the past 30 years, medication adherence theoretical approaches have primarily focused on understanding and changing the psychology of the person taking medications. Altering attitudes and beliefs are the focal concepts of these theories. The Theory of Planned Behavior has been used to examine the person's beliefs and attitudes toward medication taking.[7] According to this theory, behavior is a function of one's intention to perform the behavior. Intention is affected not only by the attitude toward medication taking but also by the individual's perceptions of how others view medication taking and the perceived amount of control the person has over medication taking.

The Social Cognitive Theory[8–11] is another popular theoretical approach. This theory proposes that behavior is affected by personal factors, such as cognitive, affective, and biologic influences, and the environment through social and physical influences. Although this theory includes both the person and the environment, the environment, as described in the theory, is only important in as much as it is cognitively and mentally understood by and through the individual.

Leventhal and colleagues'[12,13] Self-Regulation Model has also been used in several medication adherence studies.[14–16] This model proposes that health behaviors are influenced by the objective observations and emotional responses related to illness representations, perceived symptoms, and the real or perceived outcomes of health behaviors. Other psychological theories of behavior that have been used in medication adherence reports include the Theory of Reasoned Action,[17] the Health Belief Model,[18] and the PRECEDE (Predisposing, Reinforcing, Enabling, Causes in, Educational Diagnosis and Evaluation) model.[19]

Recently, the adherence theoretical scope has broadened to include theories that include systems thinking. The World Health Organization's 2003 adherence model consists of 5 interacting dimensions: patient-related factors, condition-related factors, social/economic factors, therapy-related factors, and health care system/health care team–related factors.[4] Ecological models are also now entering the field of adherence, looking at patients and their adherence behavior as being surrounded by influences at multiple levels of the community and health care system.[20]

MEDICATION ADHERENCE INTERVENTIONS

Medication adherence interventions have targeted the older adult and medication taking largely through efforts to change knowledge, attitudes and beliefs, and associated behavior.[21,22] Although most medication adherence studies do not report any theoretical underpinning, they typically attempt to enhance intention and knowledge through education (verbal, written, Internet), attitude and motivation through counseling (to change negative thoughts about medications), and associated behavior through cues, reminders, and self-monitoring.[21–23] Education and counseling are the most commonly studied approaches.[21,22] Targeted educational interventions most frequently involve providing information about medication indications, frequency, dose, side effects, and the importance of medications for illness management. Educational interventions are effective at changing knowledge but are not effective in changing medication adherence behavior.[24] Counseling often involves patient contact by a health care provider, most likely a pharmacist, nurse, or physician, for varied frequencies and lengths of time.[21] Content of counseling sessions are usually not well delineated.[25] Education and counseling are frequently combined with other interventions such as encouraging the use of cues and medication organizers and self-monitoring of medication effects.[21]

Even with multifaceted interventions, effect sizes in meta-analyses have been small.[5,26–28] Effect size is a statistical value that measures the strength of the relationship between 2 variables and allows comparison of intervention effects across studies.[29] Like correlations, effect sizes can be small (d = 0.2), medium (d = 0.5), or large (d = 0.8).[30] Examining 52 adherence studies from the general population using a meta-analytic approach, Roter and colleagues[26] found that educational interventions had an effect size of 0.13, affective interventions an effect size of 0.18, behavioral interventions an effect size of 0.20, and combined interventions an effect size of 0.24. Likewise, Peterson and colleagues[27] analyzed 23 medication adherence studies and found an educational intervention effect size of 0.11 and behavioral intervention effect size of 0.07.

Narrative review findings corroborate meta-analysis findings that limited benefits to medication adherence occur with interventions preoccupied with intention and motivation. Statistically significant improvements appear in only half of the studies, and patterns suggesting which interventions are effective have not been documented.[21,28,31,32] Haynes and colleagues[31] systematically reviewed 69 randomized controlled trial (RCT) reports, with only 36 of 81 (44%) indicating statistical significance. McDonald and colleagues[32] reviewed 33 RCTs and found only 19 of 39 (49%) showed statistically significant improvements in medication adherence. Similarly, Russell and colleagues[21] and Kripalani and colleagues[28] reviewed 57 and 37 reports, respectively, and discovered statistical significance in only 54% of the reports. Current interventions are just as likely to be ineffective as effective in improving medication adherence. If medication adherence is to be improved, we must abandon interventions focused on personal characteristics, intentional and motivation, and instead look to a more innovative approach.

A PARADIGM SHIFT

Thomas Kuhn,[33] in his book *The Structure of Scientific Revolutions*, notes that knowledge development in science does not progress in a linear or continuous manner but instead periodically goes through revolutions called paradigm shifts. During these shifts, development of a scientific field undergoes transformation.

Kuhn suggests that there are 3 stages of development of science[33]: prescience, normal science, and revolutionary science. In prescience, the field has no central paradigm, and knowledge development is rather haphazard. The next stage, normal science, involves studying and testing the theory or theories related to a particular field. No challenges to the theory or theories emerge in this phase. However, this phase is highly productive and moves the field forward. During the revolutionary science phase, findings early in this phase are contradictory to the theory or theories and are interpreted researcher problems. Because contradictory results accumulate, the field reaches a crisis. A new paradigm is born in which the normal science phase results and the revolutionary science results merge.

PERSONAL SYSTEMS APPROACH

"To Err is Human," the Institute of Medicine's landmark report on improving hospital safety, suggests moving away from blaming the individual and, instead, making the desired behavior more likely to occur by removing environmental barriers.[34] Strategies have been implemented in health care organizations not only at the level of large systems and the community to improve health care delivery but also at the personal systems level as part of the efforts to improve health outcomes.[35–38] Community health has been improved targeting personal systems processes, including improved neonatal mortality rates and decreased young adult school suspensions.[39] The intervention has been used successfully at a personal level to reduce stress,[40] lower asthma attacks,[41] improve eating behaviors,[42] increase exercise,[43] and enhance care of those with hypertension.[44]

The need for new and innovative medication adherence interventions is urgent. Evidence has suggested personal systems change as a promising behavior change intervention far superior to targeting individual characteristics, motivation, and intention.[45–47] Personal systems change is a process of systematically improving individual systems through collaboratively shaping routines, involving supportive others in routines, and using medication self-monitoring to change and maintain behavior.[48] Individual systems include the people and the daily routines that shape personal lives and activities.

Personal systems interventions are improving health behaviors. A recent systematic review of 8 personal systems intervention studies was completed.[49] The studies targeted a broad range of health outcomes. Studies addressed lifestyle changes, stress management, weight loss, increasing and maintaining exercise, improving work habits, and medication adherence. Improvements in health behavior outcomes were dramatic. The 3 reports targeting lifestyle changes in students indicated that 45% to 83% of the students reported an improvement in their individual lifestyle improvement projects.[48,50,51] Improvements were also found in medication adherence and exercise maintenance.[43,52]

The personal systems intervention for medication adherence change uses a 4-pronged patient-driven approach: (1) assessing individual systems (including important others who shape medication taking) and the system's impact on medication taking and proposing individual systems solutions to improve medication adherence, (2) implementing the proposed individual systems solutions to improve medication adherence, (3) tracking medication adherence data, and (4) evaluating medication adherence data.[53]

A brief overview of each of the key steps in this approach is presented.[48] In step 1, the person is guided by the interventionist to look beyond personal motivation to the life routines in the environment and persons who shape those routines. Daily, weekly, and monthly life routines are identified. Current and optimum medication-taking steps are delineated. The impact of these life routines on current and optimum medication taking are noted. Personal system-level solutions supporting medication adherence that tap into life routines in the individual's environment are identified.

In step 2 of the personal systems approach, the personal system-level solutions identified in step 1 are implemented to test for effectiveness. Under the guidance of the interventionist, personal system changes are incorporated into the person's life routines. The desirable behavior, in this case medication taking, is linked to routines. Routines can be adjusted to support the desired behavior. In this way, the behavior occurs because the routine occurs and not because of motivation, remembering, or effort.

Step 3 involves tracking data. Personal system-level change is facilitated by tracking data on the effectiveness of the change so that patterns can be found. Electronic medication adherence monitoring using medication event monitoring systems (MEMS; AARDEX Group, Switzerland) has been used successfully to provide individuals their medication-taking report.[52] This report, an example of which is presented in **Fig. 1**, includes the name of the medication being monitored; the range of dates for the report; general information (the number of monitored days, number of prescribed doses, number of doses taken); taking information (percentage of prescribed number of doses taken, percentage of days the number of doses taken); and hours (interdose intervals and percentage of prescribed doses taken on schedule), days (x-axis), times (y-axis), medication-taking goal (shaded horizontal bar), dots for each time the electronic monitoring cap was opened with a presumed medication ingestion, triangles for missed doses, and vertical bar when both doses are missed on a day.

Step 4 of the personal systems approach involves evaluating the data to see if a change was indeed effective. With medication taking, both dosing and timing of medications may be evaluated for goal achievement. Under the guidance of the interventionist, these processes are continued until the behavioral goal of medication adherence is achieved.

People find this personal system approach to be engaging and well accepted.[52] This technique removes blame from the medication adherence communication between the health care provider and patient. Instead, both focus on objective medication-taking data to achieve the patient's medication adherence goal.

FUTURE TRENDS IN MEDICATION ADHERENCE IN OLDER ADULTS

Testing and implementing personal systems interventions to improve medication adherence are certainly accompanied by other advances. Medication adherence guidelines for older adults are currently available for use by health care providers.[54] Publication of RCTs to test interventions to improve medication adherence in older adults has progressively increased over the past few decades.[21] Concomitantly, the number of meta-analyses and medication adherence guidelines are also growing.[24,55] Medication adherence assessment and intervention guidelines have been developed into pocket-sized versions to enhance ease of use by health care practitioners.[56] However, given that many of these guidelines have developed from evidence that shows limited effectiveness in improving medication adherence, these guidelines

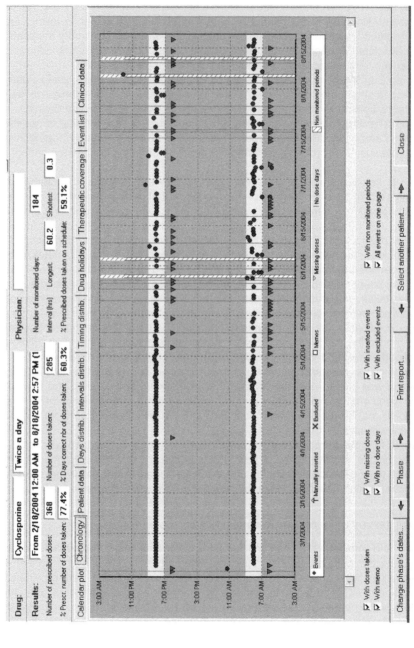

Fig. 1. Medication event monitoring systems report for tracking medication adherence data.

may not have the desired impact. Medication adherence guideline effectiveness evaluation studies have not been systematically conducted. Funding sources are available for performing translational research studies to determine guideline effectiveness. We welcome these study results. Findings from these studies may add clarity to the problem of the need for more innovative approaches to medication adherence interventions.

Technology will affect the future of medication adherence interventions with older adults. Health information technology links health care providers, health care consumers, and information.[57] This powerful technology assists health care providers in securely managing medical information.[57] Technology, including medication adherence technology, has the potential to improve health care quality, prevent medical errors, increase care efficiency, reduce unnecessary health care costs, decrease paperwork, and improve population health.[57] Medication adherence data can be gathered, processed, and delivered to both patients and providers in a timely, secure, and accurate manner through electronic medication-monitoring systems.[52] Wireless medication-monitoring systems will soon be available to enhance this exchange. Technology firms are developing wearable devices that have the potential to monitor the behavior of medication ingestion as well as other biological parameters. Decision-support information, such as electronic medication-monitoring data "provides clinicians, staff, patients, or other individuals with knowledge and person-specific information, intelligently filtered or presented at appropriate times to enhance health and health care."[57(para1)] Technology to improve health care behaviors has focused on self-monitoring, cueing health care behaviors, and providing education and support delivered via the computer or Internet.[52,58–62] Results are encouraging. Tremendous potential exists to further refine and enhance decision-support information related to medication adherence.

Several other advances in medications are likely to affect medication adherence. Pharmacogenomics, or the tailoring of medications to an individual's genetic makeup, may allow lower doses of medications to be used, which could increase the efficiency of medication delivery and decrease medication side effects. Fixed-dose medication delivery, which delivers multiple medications in a single dose, may greatly decrease the number of pills that must be taken. Decreased medication-dosing frequency, which changes the number of times that a medication must be taken to be effective, is also a future improvement. Medication dosing is changing from multiple dosing per day to weekly, monthly, or yearly dosing.

SUMMARY

We review the theories and interventions used to attempt improvement in older adults' medication adherence behavior. Using Kuhn's model, we propose a paradigm shift in behavior change intervention toward a novel medication adherence intervention that focuses on tapping into the personal system in which the individual functions to change medication-taking behavior that moves away from focusing on personal characteristics, motivation, and intention. We discuss the evidence that has tested this personal systems approach We also discuss future trends in research and practice with medication adherence in older adults. Medication nonadherence is a prevalent and perplexing problem in older adults. We anticipate the problem to increase both in prevalence and complexity in the future. Adherence intervention research has been languishing with modest results for more than 30 years. Clinicians are frustrated by their inability to offer patients effective medication adherence interventions. Patients are tired of being blamed for medication nonadherence. There is a need for a paradigm shift from focusing on characteristics, motivation, and intention of the patients to the personal systems in which patients live their daily life while also taking into account the needed changes in health care systems and health policy.

REFERENCES

1. The Department of Health and Human Services Division of Aging. 2010. Available at: http://www.aoa.gov/aoaroot/aging_statistics/index.aspx. Accessed December 15, 2010.
2. Centers for Disease Control and Prevention. 2010. Available at: http://www.cdc.gov/chronicdisease/overview/index.htm. Accessed December 30, 2010.
3. Dunbar-Jacob J, Erlen JA, Schlenk EA, et al. Adherence in chronic disease. Annu Rev Nurs Res 2000;18:48–90.
4. Sabate E. Adherence to long-term therapies: evidence for action. Geneva (Switzerland): World Health Organization; 2003.
5. Schlenk EA, Dunbar-Jacob J, Engberg S. Medication non-adherence among older adults: a review of strategies and interventions for improvement. J Gerontol Nurs 2004;30(7):33–43.
6. Di Matteo MR. Variations in patients' adherence to medical recommendations: a quantitative review of 50 years of research. Med Care 2004;42(3):200–9.
7. Ajzen I, Fishbein M. Understanding attitudes and predicting social behavior. Englewood Cliffs (NJ): Prentice-Hall; 1980.
8. Russell CL, Conn V, Ashbaugh C, et al. Medication adherence patterns in adult renal transplant recipients. Res Nurs Health 2006;29(6):521–32.
9. Russell CL, Cetingok M, Hamburger KQ, et al. Medication adherence in older renal transplant recipients. Clin Nurs Res 2010;19(2):95–112.
10. Friedman RH. Automated telephone conversations to assess health behavior and deliver behavioral interventions. J Med Syst 1998;22(2):95–102.
11. Bandura A. Health promotion from the perspective of social cognitive theory. In: Norman P, editor. Understanding and changing health behavior: from health beliefs to self-regulation. United Kingdom: Psychology Press; 2000. p. 299–339.
12. Leventhal H, Nerenz DR, Straus A. Self-regulation and the mechanisms for symptom appraisal. In: Mechanic D, editor. Symptoms, illness behavior, and help-seeking. New York: Prodist; 1982. p. 55–86.
13. Leventhal H, Zimmerman R, Gutmann M. Compliance: a self-regulation perspective. In: Gentry WD, editor. Handbook of behavioral medicine. New York: Guilford Press; 1984. p. 369–436.
14. Ross S, Walker A, MacLeod MJ. Patient compliance in hypertension: role of illness perceptions and treatment beliefs. J Hum Hypertens 2004;18:607–13.
15. Ruppar TM. Randomized pilot study of a behavioral feedback intervention to improve medication adherence in older adults with hypertension. J Cardiovasc Nurs 2010;25(6):470–9.
16. Horne R, Weinman J. Self-regulation and self-management in asthma: exploring the role of illness perceptions and treatment beliefs in explaining non-adherence to prevent medication. Psychology & Health 2002;17(1):17.
17. Halfmann SM. Peer support with a nurse-managed intervention and compliance after a cardiac event, vol. 138. Denton (TX): Texas Woman's University; 2000. **PhD.
18. Conner M, Norman P. Predicting health behavior. Search and practice with social cognition models. Ballman (Buckingham): Open University Press Buckingham; 1996.

19. Robbins B, Rausch KJ, Garcia RI, et al. Multicultural medication adherence: a comparative study. J Gerontol Nurs 2004;30(7):25–32.
20. McLeroy KR, Bibeau D, Steckler A, et al. An ecological perspective on health promotion programs. Health Educ Q 1988;15(4):351–77.
21. Russell CL, Conn V, Jantarakupt P. Older adult medication compliance: integrated review of randomized controlled trials. Am J Health Behav 2006;30: 636–50.
22. Schlenk EA, Bernardo LM, Organist LA, et al. Optimizing medication adherence in older patients: a systematic review. J Clin Outcomes Manag 2008;15(12): 595–606.
23. Ruppar T, Conn V, Russell CL. Medication adherence interventions for older adults: a literature review. Res Theory Nurs Pract 2008;22(2):114–47.
24. Conn VS, Hafdahl AR, Cooper P, et al. Interventions to improve medication adherence among older adults: meta-analysis of adherence outcomes among randomized controlled trials. Gerontologist 2009;49:447–62.
25. Conn VS, Cooper PS, Ruppar TM, et al. Searching for the intervention in intervention research reports. J Nurs Scholarsh 2008;40(1):52–9.
26. Roter DL, Hall JA, Merisca R, et al. Effectiveness of interventions to improve patient compliance: a meta-analysis. Med Care 1998;36(8):1138–61.
27. Peterson AM, Takiya L, Finley R. Meta-analysis of trials of interventions to improve medication adherence. Am J Health Syst Pharm 2003;60:657–65.
28. Kripalani S, Yao X, Haynes RB. Interventions to enhance medication adherence in chronic conditions. Arch Intern Med 2007;167:540–50.
29. Cohen J. Statistical power analysis in the behavioral sciences. Hillsdale (NJ): Erlbaum; 1988.
30. Tucker CM, Desmond FF, Cohen JL, et al. Nurses' attitudes, nurse-patient interactions and adherence to treatment by hemodialysis patients. Psychol Rep 1991; 68(3 Pt 1):733–4.
31. Haynes RB, Yao X, Degani A, et al. Interventions for enhancing medication adherence [systematic review]. Cochrane Database Syst Rev 2005;4:CD000011.
32. McDonald HP, Garg AX, Haynes RB. Interventions to enhance patient adherence to medication prescriptions. JAMA 2002;288(22):2868–79.
33. Kuhn T. The structure of scientific revolutions. Chicago (IL): The University of Chicago Press; 1962.
34. Kohn KT, Corrigan JM, Donaldson MS. To err is human: building a safer health system. Washington, DC: National Academy Press; 1999.
35. Harrigan S, Hurst D, Lee C, et al. Developing and implementing quality initiatives in the ICU: strategies and outcomes. Crit Care Nurs Clin North Am 2006;18(4): 469–79.
36. Imperiali G, Minoli G, Meucci GM, et al. Effectiveness of a continuous quality improvement program on colonoscopy practice. Endoscopy 2007;39(4):314–8.
37. Jain M, Miller L, Belt D, et al. Decline in ICU adverse events, nosocomial infections and cost through a quality improvement initiative focusing on teamwork and culture change. Qual Saf Health Care 2006;15(4):235–9.
38. Potisek NM, Malone RM, Shilliday BB, et al. Use of patient flow analysis to improve patient visit efficiency by decreasing wait time in a primary care-based disease management programs for anticoagulation and chronic pain: a quality improvement study. BMC Health Services Research 2007;7:8.
39. Knapp M, Hotopp D. Applying TQM to community health improvement: nine works in progress [erratum appears in Qual Lett Healthc Lead 1995 Sep;7(7):15]. Qual Lett Healthc Lead 1995;7(6):23–9.

40. Lundeen E, Pai-Fisher E, Neuhauser D. Continuous self improvement to reduce stress: developing an individualized model of health. Qual Manag Health Care 2001;9(3):47–56.
41. Alemi F, Neuhauser D. Time-between control charts for monitoring asthma attacks. Jt Comm Qual Saf 2004;30(2):95–102.
42. Alemi F, Pawloski L, Fallon WF Jr. System thinking in a personal context to improve eating behaviors. J Healthc Qual 2003;25(2):20–5.
43. Moore S, Charvat J. Using the CHANGE intervention to enhance long-term exercise. Nurs Clin North Am 2002;37(2):272–83.
44. Hebert C, Neuhauser D. Improving hypertension care with patient-generated run charts: physician, patient, and management perspectives. Qual Manag Health Care 2004;13(3):174–7.
45. De Geest S, Dobbels F, Fluri C, et al. Adherence to the therapeutic regimen in heart, lung, and heart-lung transplant recipients. J Cardiol Nurs 2005;20(Suppl 5): S88–98.
46. Denhaerynck K, Dobbels F, Cleemput I, et al. Prevalence, consequences, and determinants of nonadherence in adult renal transplant patients: a literature review. Transpl Int 2005;18(10):1121–33.
47. Desmyttere A, Dobbels F, Cleemput I, et al. Noncompliance with immunosuppressive regimen in organ transplantation: is it worth worrying about? Acta Gastroenterol Belg 2005;68(3):347–52.
48. Alemi F, Neuhauser D, Ardito S, et al. Continuous self-improvement: systems thinking in a personal context. Jt Comm J Qual Improv 2000;26(2):74–86.
49. Matteson MM, Russell CL. Systematic review of continuous self-improvement interventions 2011.
50. Bacon DR, Stewart KA. The personal data analysis exercise. J Manag Educ 2001; 25(1):70–8.
51. Kyrkjebo JM, Hanestad BR. Personal improvement project in nursing education: learning methods and tools for continuous quality improvement in nursing practice. J Adv Nurs 2003;41(1):88–98.
52. Russell CL, Conn VS, Ashbaugh C, et al. Taking immunosuppressive medications effectively (TIMELink): a pilot randomized controlled trial in adult kidney transplant recipients. Clin Transplant 2010.
53. Russell CL. A clinical nurse specialist-led intervention to enhance medication adherence using the plan-do-check-act cycle for continuous self-improvement. Clin Nurse Spec 2010;24:69–75.
54. Zwicker D, Fulmer T. Reducing adverse drug events. In: Capezuti E, Zwicker D, Mezey M, et al, editors. Evidence-based geriatric nursing protocols for best practice. 3rd edition. New York: Springer Publishing Company, Inc; 2008. p. 257–308.
55. Medicines adherence: involving patients in decisions about prescribed medicines and supporting adherence. London: National Health Service: National Institute for Health and Clinical Excellence; 2009.
56. Transplant360. 2010; Available at: http://www.transplant360.com/. Accessed December 18, 2010.
57. Department of Health and Human Services. Health Information Technology. 2010. Available at: http://healthit.hhs.gov. Accessed June 18, 2010.
58. Schaefer-Keller P, Dickenmann M, Berry D, et al. Computer-assisted patient education in kidney transplantation: testing the content validity and usability of the Organ Transplant Information System (OTIS). Patient Educ Couns 2009;74: 110–7.

59. Russell CL, Owens S, Hamburger K, et al. Medication adherence and older renal transplant patients' perceptions of electronic medication event monitoring. J Gerontol Nurs 2009;35(10):17–21.

60. Dew MA, Goycoolea JM, Harris RC, et al. An Internet-based intervention to improve psychosocial outcomes in heart transplant recipients and family caregivers: development and evaluation. J Heart Lung Transplant 2004;23(6):745–58.

61. De Geest S, Schaefer-Keller P, Denhaerynck K, et al. Supporting medication adherence in renal transplantation (SMART): a pilot RCT to improve adherence to immunosuppressive regimens. Clin Transplant 2006;20:359–68.

62. Miloh T, Annunziato R, Arnon R, et al. Improved adherence and outcomes for pediatric liver transplant recipients by using text messaging. Pediatrics 2009; 124(5):e844–50.

Ethics of Patient Education and How Do We Make it Everyone's Ethics

Barbara K. Redman, PhD, MBE[a,b,*]

KEYWORDS

- Patient self-management • Ethics • Chronic disease
- Patient education

Patient education has long been central to nursing's philosophy of practice, and, because of this commitment, we have been deeply distressed with the cavalier and generally incomplete manner in which it is practiced in the health care system. This article focuses on the ethical underpinning of this distress and of this neglect of patient education and what nurses can do to right this wrong.

The Code of Ethics for Nurses describes the nurse's duty to advocate for and strive to protect the health, safety, and rights of the patient, with the primary commitment being to the patient.[1] A prominent bioethicist describes the primary goal of the social institution of morality to promote human flourishing by counteracting conditions that cause the quality of people's lives to worsen. Beauchamp[2] also describes a condition of culturally induced moral ignorance in which cultural factors prevent individuals from discerning what they are morally required to do. These statements characterize the dilemma facing nurses: education is clearly essential to patient safety and flourishing; nursing's code of ethics makes such practice a duty; and, yet, the dominant culture of medicine, which drives allocation of resources and privileges, pays only lip service to patient education.

Evidence of incomplete education, potentially endangering patients, is every-where—at hospital discharge, in emergency rooms, and in persons with chronic disease needing to self-manage their disease control regimen and make lifestyle changes. Evidence of the effectiveness and crucial nature of patient education is also readily available. For example, accuracy and safety of cancer chemotherapy has become urgent as patients administer their own oral regimens at home, using agents that carry side effects and narrow therapeutic ranges. Safety and prescription errors can occur unnoticed, especially because many patients believe such treatment

[a] Wayne State University, College of Nursing, 5557 Cass Avenue, Detroit, MI 48202, USA
[b] Center for Bioethics, University of Pennsylvania, Philadelphia, PA 19104-3308, USA
* Wayne State University, College of Nursing, 5557 Cass Avenue, Detroit, MI 48202.
E-mail address: ae9080@wayne.edu

Nurs Clin N Am 46 (2011) 283–289
doi:10.1016/j.cnur.2011.05.001
0029-6465/11/$ – see front matter © 2011 Elsevier Inc. All rights reserved.

has minimal, if any, side effects, and patients need to recognize extreme side effects and stop the drug.[3]

In a second example of greatly increasing patient self-management (PSM), persons with Parkinson disease must self-monitor reemergence of symptoms associated with long-term treatment with dopaminergic therapy (called wearing off). The first symptoms to reemerge are neither well established nor the same for all patients, and wearing off is underrecognized in clinical practice. Patients must promptly recognize symptoms and their relationship to the next dose, to trigger dose adjustment or adjunctive therapy, to optimize long-term benefits.[4]

Additional examples of increased patient responsibility are legion. What are we to do about the disconnect between obvious benefits from patient education and ethical standards that would seem to require its provision for human flourishing and the current state of sloppy incomplete delivery? How do we deal with culturally induced moral ignorance (high-technology treatment locking) in which interlocking forces and cultural norms, including reimbursement systems, training programs, and physician dominance, tremendously inhibit meeting patients' low-technology human needs for basic education to keep them safe?

What are the chances of reforming the system? Because dominant players in health policy (read doctors and hospitals) lose dramatically in a shift to a balanced portfolio of services patients need rather than those they wish to provide, these players resist, leaving unexamined the very real costs of not changing the system. The greatest effort to achieve this reform is being played out in the United Kingdom's National Health Service through its Expert Patient Initiative in which those with chronic illness are educated and supported in PSM. Part of the incentive is to control health care costs, which can, at the same time, improve patient care.

Part of the cultural moral ignorance related to patient education also extends to bioethics. For example, although the doctrine of informed consent seems to be friendly to assuring patient understanding, frequent disclosure of information to patients or research subjects is all that is required. There is a false assumption that disclosure automatically leads to understanding with no assistance. Evidence of incomplete patient understanding has led to questions about whether informed consent is an achievable norm. The answer, of course, is that it likely is, if the norm includes definition of appropriate education to help patients reach understanding. The author has served on multiple hospital ethics committees. In none of them has the question of inadequate patient education been defined as problematic, consumed as these committees often are, with questions of end of life.

To explore underlying ethical issues, this article is divided into 3 parts: (1) 3 crucial questions to account for the current state of affairs; (2) alternative systems by which patient education could be delivered, including ethical ideals for any such system; and (3) recommendations for next steps.

3 CRUCIAL QUESTIONS

Although crucial from pragmatic and ethical perspectives, none of the following 3 questions has been adequately explored:

1. What kinds of ends (outcomes) for patient education best serve the patient's needs?
   The mantra of the discipline of health education has long been that changes in health behaviors are the only appropriate outcome, frequently along the lines of compliance with the medical regimen. Elsewhere, the author[5] has explored the

moral framework of development of capabilities, especially as described by Nussbaum,[6] as more appropriate. Capabilities developing what people are able to do or be are guaranteed to a threshold level. People to whom patient education can most contribute include those being able to think and reason, to develop emotion, to engage in critical reflection about the planning of one's life, and to live with others. Such a framework links education of patients to all kinds of life education and avoids capture by narrow medical thinking.

Recent PSM programs have been oriented to problem solving, action planning, goal setting, dealing with difficult emotions, healthy living, medication and symptom management, and working in partnership with health professionals.[7] This orientation is much closer to a capabilities approach than is the typical compliance-with-medical-regimen orientation and acknowledges that skills learned are transferable to other areas of life and leads to another question.

2. How closely should patient education be tethered to a physician's orders?
A previous assumption that lack of tight tethering to the physician's treatment plan constituted subordination is gradually giving way to an assumption that there is a body of evidence about what patients should know and be able to do, which is separate from and should be able to override an individual physician's view. In addition, the quality of care provided by individual physician practitioners is fraught with clinical inertia (seeing patients but not adjusting regimen to yield appropriate outcomes) and outright poor practice, making patient understanding and ability to care for oneself an important element of safety.

Nurses responsible for patient education frequently report ethical conflicts with physicians over authority to dictate what patients are taught. Perhaps, when real team-based care, in which one member can challenge another, is practiced, the situation may be different.

3. Why is patient education so incompletely practiced, and what can be done about it?
Although the cultural and structural issues outlined earlier are important, once again the United Kingdom is leading the way. Within a national quality improvement program for self-management of long-term conditions, clinicians are offered training to enhance their sense of competence and confidence to effectively deliver PSM support services. Although PSM requires patients to be activated, informed, and empowered, the support of clinicians who are willing to work in partnership with their patients to develop mutually accepted and followed treatment plans is also needed. Skills in collaborative goal setting and follow-up and ability to respect the patient's choice are part of such training.[8]

The focus here, rather than other questions pertinent to the ethics of patient education, is perhaps the most hypocritical—we say that patient education is available in the health care system, but for many this is not true. Other ethical issues deserving of discussion include lack of professional standards of practice and availability of a cluster of highly predictive measurement instruments, to be developed elsewhere.

ALTERNATIVE SYSTEMS BY WHICH PATIENT EDUCATION FOR PSM COULD BE DELIVERED

An important part of ethical analysis involves examination of benefits and harms from alternatives. Chronic disease, even in its acute exacerbations, is very common and requires sustained support from a reliable system of care. Alternative systems for delivery of PSM preparation and support should be examined. It is easy to think of such alternatives, but, initially, it is useful to lay out ideals against which any proposed system could be judged.

These ideals might include

- Patients can do as much PSM as they want and are capable of doing, with both preferences and competencies documented at intervals in the course of a chronic disease because they do change. Payment or resource allocation rules under which health systems operate may push toward more PSM because it is believed, in the long run, to be more cost effective and frequently to assure better outcomes (hypertension, anticoagulation).
- Benefits from patient education are optimized and harms minimized and contained. Benefits include better care, placing the disease in perspective with other life goals, and learning PSM skills transferable to other areas of life. Potential harms from patient education and PSM are rarely monitored in research or practice but include mistakes in caring for oneself or others and guilt and shame from inability to control the course of a disease.[9]
- PSM should not be dependent on literacy, numeracy, or formal educational level. Low health literacy is a strong predictor of poor health outcomes. Incorrect disease-related beliefs may be one of the pathways through which health literacy influences health outcomes. For example, older adults with asthma and inadequate health literacy were significantly more likely to have beliefs about asthma that are associated with poor asthma control, including the no-symptom-no-asthma belief, the belief that asthma is curable and the belief that asthma controller medications work better if they are not used all the time. Interventions to correct such beliefs are part of PSM support and should be used in conjunction with low literacy interventions.[10]
- Treatment decisions and their rationale should be transparent to the patient and to other team members and open to regular feedback and correction.

Against these ideals, there are at least 3 alternative models for delivery of patient education services, which can be considered. The first is improvement in the current professional practice model, making norms for adequate PSM support clear and delivering first feedback and then zingers to practitioners who do not meet them. Such an approach requires coordinated activity among payers and/or accreditors, although the latter are primarily focused on inpatient care and not on outpatient settings where most chronic illness care is delivered. Development of better safety and quality indicators for outpatient care is necessary. The Chronic Disease Self Management Program pioneered by Lorig and others[7] has in the United Kingdom been integrated into the health care system but in the United States stands outside it, independently sponsored by community organizations and not requiring a provider referral. But such programs are of short term and clearly cannot create relationships that last the life of the illness as a good provider-patient relationship can.

The second model would likely horrify many health professionals, that is, providing patient education and PSM support on the open market, with regulation to keep it free of fraud and deception. What we forget is that health care in the United States is already heavily market focused and arguably still has not attained the safety and efficacy that are supposed to follow from a well-functioning market. Under a market model, organizations providing patient education services compete based on quality of care. Payment (from whatever source) is tied to performance and patient satisfaction, with patients free to vote with their feet.

Market values predominate, perhaps altered by soft paternalism to counteract people's well-documented proclivity to not understand statistics and to use unconscious behaviors that cause them to act against their own best interests.[11] PSM would always be required (the default), with adequate safety testing and support, unless persons with chronic illness opted out. Such support helps people understand the accuracy of their ability to sense their bodily state and think through their preferences, understanding that people are imperfect decision makers.

The third model (public health) has been tried with diabetes and, potentially, other chronic diseases in New York City. The public health authority began tracking (through laboratory reports of HbA1C) quality of outcomes being attained by physicians and their patients with diabetes, with feedback to both. Public health approaches have most frequently been associated with control of infectious diseases but could easily be extended to chronic diseases, which are also a major threat to the public's health.

The public health system does not seem to be a reliable provider of direct health care services or even a monitor of the outcomes of chronic care services. Some believe that public health should be limited to its official legal functions. Although health equity is a central value of public health systems, these programs are population based and often compulsory and may not be beneficial to each individual person.[12] Whether public health systems can make the transition from a focus predominantly on communicable disease to encompass what it means to live well as one ages with a chronic disease is open to question.[13] Although such a move requires wide public discussion, such a forum might be the best way to develop a new set of norms to replace notions of decay and sickness common in current discussions of chronic disease.

It is possible that all 3 models could operate simultaneously because they are on a small scale now. But without some common level of definition of safety and acceptable quality of care and a means of enforcement, these systems remain very partial and, in the aggregate, unsatisfactory.

RECOMMENDATIONS FOR NEXT STEPS

What can nurses on the front line of practice in all settings do to put patient education in its rightful place, thus better serving patients and decreasing the ethical distress that often follow inability to practice to appropriate standards? It is important to note that what we are really about is changing the norms of care. Do not expect it to be linear or smooth; just keep up the pressure points.

There are several steps that the profession, often in conjunction with patient and family advocacy groups, can take to change the moral and operating norms around patient competency to undertake their own care.

1. Roles for certified educators are well established in diabetes care and being established in respiratory care. In Canada, Certified Respiratory Educators provide patient education with emphasis on PSM, instruction in proper inhaler technique, and advice to patients about their asthma or chronic obstructive pulmonary disease and on how to deal with exacerbations.[14]
2. Nurses regularly serve in other roles in which the importance of patient education can be reinforced. These include roles in safety and quality assurance and in institutional ethics committees. Much chronic disease care occurs in ambulatory settings, an area where little patient safety research and safety improvement work has been accomplished. Outpatient settings are often fragmented, lacking systems of accountability for locating errors, correcting them, and developing

systems to increase safety. One such approach is patients' access to their own electronic medical records, fortified with patient education so that they can interpret test results, catch medication errors, and be their own safety monitor.[15] This kind of safeguard may favor the most educated and certainly should not substitute for professional systems of safety improvement.

3. Nurses in many areas of practice must play advocacy roles in changing the system to make patients safer through patient education. Oncology and the rapidly evolving use of oral chemotherapy can be taken as an example. Since 2005, at least 10 oral chemotherapy medications have been introduced into the market. Many people incorrectly believe that these medications are less toxic than intravenous chemotherapy; yet, most insurance companies, including Medicare, do not reimburse for nursing time spent on educating patients how to safely take these medications. A model for such a nursing role is well described by Moody and Jackowski.[16]

Another example occurs with anticoagulant therapy. In some European countries, PSM of this therapy is well established because it increases the time when the patient is in the therapeutic range and thus decreases adverse events. But in other countries, this therapy, used for protection against stroke in patients with atrial fibrillation or mechanical valve replacement or management of venous thromboembolism, is not optimally practiced. An interview study of patients and their physicians in Australia showed lack of practitioner awareness of patient difficulties and very little patient education at commencement of anticoagulant therapy. (It should be noted that this study oversampled patients with an episode of significant overcoagulation, thus likely high risk.) Development of a nursing role to optimize this therapy is suggested.[17] Such clinical examples are legion, and their number is increasing rapidly. The opportunity to develop and advocate for these roles must be taken and the difference they make in patient outcomes documented.

SUMMARY

Make no mistake; forcing new norms supporting patient education takes concerted effort from nurses practicing everywhere. We need to be clear about why this change is urgent (patient safety and satisfaction), what is an appropriate end goal (patient capabilities to make health a part of their lived life), and that patient education should be available in all practice settings, delivered through clinical, market, and public health models, most effectively in some sort of national structure as in the United Kingdom's Expert Patient Program. Most of all, we need to get rid of outdated ideas such as patient education depends on the physician's permission or treatment plan; adherence to the medical regimen is the prime outcome goal (it is extremely important in some situations but as part of a broader set of goals); or insurers, administrators, and others in authority will gratefully support patient education when the need is pointed out to them (they will resist it because it is not central to the medical model around which they entire health care system is structured).

Yet, patient education ought to be thought of as basic to ethical practice and the lack of it as a form of abandonment.

REFERENCES

1. American Nurses Association. Code of ethics for nurses. Washington, DC: American Nurses Association; 2001.
2. Beauchamp TL. Standing principles. New York: Oxford University Press; 2010.

3. Halfdanarson TR, Jatoi A. Oral cancer chemotherapy: the critical interplay between patient education and patient safety. Curr Oncol Rep 2010;12:247–52.

4. Stacy M. The wearing-off phenomenon and the use of questionnaires to facilitate its recognition in Parkinson's disease. J Neural Transm 2010;117:837–46.

5. Redman BK. When is patient education unethical? Nurs Ethics 2008;15:813–20.

6. Nussbaum MC. Women and human development: the capabilities approach. Cambridge (UK): Cambridge University Press; 2000.

7. Lorig K, Holman HR, Sobel D, et al. Living a healthy life with chronic, conditions. 3rd edition. Boulder (CO): Bull Publishing; 2006.

8. Kosmala-Anderson JP, Wallace LM, Turner A. Confidence matters: a Self-Determination Theory study of factors determining engagement in self-management support practices of UK clinicians. Psychol Health Med 2010;15:478–91.

9. Redman BK. Patient self-management: potential harms to control. Chronic Illn 2010;6:151–3.

10. Federman AD, Wisnivesky JP, Wolf MS, et al. Inadequate health literacy is associated with suboptimal health beliefs in older asthmatics. J Asthma 2010;47:620–6.

11. Ubel P. Free market madness. Cambridge (MA): Harvard Business Press; 2010.

12. Dawson A, Verweij M, editors. Ethics, prevention and public health. New York: Oxford University Press; 2007.

13. Jennings B. Public health and civic republicanism. In: Dawson A, Verweij M, editors. Ethics, prevention and public health. New York: Oxford University Press; 2007. p. 30–58.

14. Field SK, Conley DP, Thawer AM, et al. Assessment and management of patients with chronic cough by Certified Respiratory Educators. Can Respir J 2009;16(2):49–54.

15. Ghandi TK, Lee TH. Patient safety beyond the hospital. N Engl J Med 2010;363:1001–3.

16. Moody M, Jackowski J. Are patients on oral chemotherapy in your practice setting safe? Clin J Oncol Nurs 2010;14:339–46.

17. Lowthian JA, Diug BO, Evans SM, et al. Who is responsible for the care of patients treated with warfarin therapy? Med J Aust 2009;190(12):674–7.

Using a Competency-Based Approach to Patient Education: Achieving Congruence Among Learning, Teaching and Evaluation

Whei Ming Su, MA, RN, CCRN[a],*, Bobbi Herron, MS, ACNS-BC[a],
Paul J. Osisek, MEd, CAGS, MS[b]

KEYWORDS

- Patient education • Competency-based education
- Chronic health problems

Millions of Americans are living with and managing their chronic health problems. Patient education plays an essential role in promoting safe self-management practice. To ensure that patients attain the required abilities, patient education needs to be competency-based. When developing and applying a competency-based patient education lesson/program, each nurse must answer questions concerning essential competencies, optimal teaching methods, best method to evaluate patient achievement, and documentation of evidence. This article describes how the authors used these questions as a guide to achieve congruence among intended learning, instruction, and evaluation to design and implement a patient education program, Managing Heart Failure, at a local hospital.

Millions of Americans are living with and managing their chronic health problems. Patient education plays an essential role in promoting safe self-management practice. The Joint Commission on the Accreditation of Health Care Organizations

The authors have nothing to disclose.
[a] Department of Nursing, Purdue University North Central, 1401 South US 421, Westville, IN 46391, USA
[b] Department of Social Science, Purdue University North Central, 1401 South US 421, Westville, IN 46391, USA
* Corresponding author.
E-mail address: wmingsu@pnc.edu

Nurs Clin N Am 46 (2011) 291–298
doi:10.1016/j.cnur.2011.05.003
0029-6465/11/$ – see front matter. Published by Elsevier Inc.

(JCAHO) mandates that each patient receive education and training specific to the patient's needs and as appropriate to the care, treatment, and services provided.[1] To meet accountability criteria, nurses not only need to document that teaching activities have taken place, but also provide evidence that learning has occurred. Verbalized understanding is often used by nurses to document actual learning outcomes of patient education. However, that phrase is not sufficient to indicate the accuracy/ degree of understanding, and to support the contention that patients are able to apply the knowledge and skills required for taking care of themselves.

To ensure that patients attain the required abilities, patient education needs to be competency-based. The main focus of competency-based education is on the outcomes; the patient education process must begin with the outcomes in mind.[2] This implies that instructional activities and evaluation methods must be carefully aligned with the intended learning outcome objectives.[2,3] Incongruence among learning outcome objectives, instruction, and evaluation may lead to the following problems:

Inability to achieve the intended learning results if the instructional activities are not aligned with the objectives

Inability to obtain sufficient evidence of teaching effectiveness if the instructional activities are not aligned with the assessment methods

Inability to provide evidence of learners' accomplishment of objectives if the assessment methods are not aligned with the objectives.[3]

When developing and applying a competency-based patient education lesson/ program, each nurse must answer the following questions:

What are the essential competencies for patient self-management of health?
What teaching methods will yield the intended learning?
What are the most appropriate methods to evaluate how well a patient has achieved the competencies?
How should the evidence of learning be documented?[2,3]

In this article, the authors describe how they used these questions as a guide to achieve congruence among intended learning, instruction, and evaluation to design and implement a patient education program, Managing Heart Failure, at a local hospital.

WHAT ARE THE ESSENTIAL COMPETENCIES FOR SELF-MANAGEMENT OF HEART FAILURE?

When determining competencies for self-management of health, patient educators must adopt current best practices. Based on the guidelines established by the American College of Cardiology (ACC) and the American Heart Association (AHA), the heart failure (HF) education nurse identified the following essential content knowledge for HF: the disease process and symptom monitoring, medication adherence, dietary adherence, and activity/exercise modification.[4]

The ultimate purpose for this education program was to prepare patients for the transfer of knowledge into real-life application. To promote transfer, learners must be engaged in cognitive processes beyond remembering.[3] In addition to remembering what was learned, learning outcome objectives need to reflect higher-order cognitive processes associated with comprehending, applying, analyzing, and evaluating.

These processes were incorporated into the learning outcome objectives for this patient education program. They are listed below:

Objective 1. Explain disease process and signs/symptoms of worsening HF
Objective 2. Differentiate expected responses from undesirable responses to medications
Objective 3. Select appropriate foods based on a prescribed diet
Objective 4. Self-critique implementation of the activity/exercise modification plan.

WHAT TEACHING METHODS WILL YIELD THE INTENDED LEARNING?

To select instructional methods that reflect the cognitive processes stated in the learning outcome objectives, patient educators need to ask, "How can I engage this patient in these specific thought processes?" Based on this analysis, the HF education nurse selected the following instructional activities:

Objective 1 involves comprehending conceptual knowledge. Examples and visual display facilitate understanding of conceptual knowledge.[3,5,6] The HF education nurse used concrete examples, graphics, and reading materials written in layman's terms to explain the pathophysiological process and signs and symptoms of worsening HF.

Objective 2 was designed to develop the patient's ability to differentiate relevant data while monitoring effects of drug therapy. Instructional activities focused on developing the patient's ability to analyze cause–effect relationships. It may be difficult for some to conceptualize the abstract thought process of analysis. Providing opportunities for learner practice in situational scenarios facilitates development of this higher-order cognitive skill.[3,5] In this case, the HF education nurse first introduced drug actions/side effects at the HF patient education class. After the introduction, she modeled by thinking aloud how to distinguish relationships among a set of clinical data related to drug therapy in a scenario. Within small groups, the patients then practiced with similar scenarios.

Objective 3 was designed to develop the patient's ability to apply principles of planning low-sodium meals. Patients were expected to compare sodium content from multiple options, choose foods with the lowest sodium content, and calculate the total amount of sodium for the foods selected. According to Benner and colleagues, Suter and Suter, and Gaberson and Oermann,[7–9] learning is enhanced when it is applied to a meaningful context. Written case studies, role playing, and simulations provide contextual meaning to learners and facilitate application of knowledge.[2,5,9,10] A grocery shopping simulation was designed as the final part of the instruction. The HF Education Nurse began with didactic presentation on sodium components of common foods and how to calculate the amount of sodium for daily meals. After the presentation, patients were asked to walk to a table where they found groups of foods, arranged to look like a shelf in a grocery store. They each had a basket and bought the lowest sodium food choices needed to prepare their sample meals. The HF education nurse guided patients to select items from a choice of meats, vegetables, breads, condiments, desserts, and drinks and to calculate the amount of sodium from the foods they selected.

Objective 4 was designed to engage patients in modifying behavior. To change behaviors, learners must perceive relevance. Reflection activities help learners make personal interpretations about their experiences and gain new insights for improving performance.[3,6,11,12] The HF education nurse conducted individual interviews with each patient before discharge. During the interview, the HF education nurse guided patients to assess their usual home activity/exercise level and reflect on how the activity level impacted their quality of life. They extended the reflection to make a plan for change. An example of this instructional interview follows.

HF education nurse: "Mr. S, what was your activity level before you came to the hospital?"

Mr. S.: "I mostly sat in the chair, because I got so short of breath when walking."

HF education nurse: "How far are you able to walk?"

Mr. S.: "I can walk to the bathroom and into the kitchen. I can't walk out into the yard, because I lose my breath."

HF education nurse: "Do you have a special event coming up that you would like to attend?" "If you could go anywhere without getting too short of breath, where would that be?"

Mr. S.: "My grandson is going to graduate from college in Florida, and I would like to have enough energy to be able to see him graduate."

HF education nurse: "What do you think you would have to do to get to that point, assuming that you get over this episode of HF?"

Mr. S.: "I would have to be able to walk through an airport, get in and out of the car, walk to the college and then to the stadium, back to the car and then back through the airport again. I need to build up my strength."

HF education nurse: "Very good. Now, how do you think we can get you that strong in the time remaining?"

Mr. S: "I don't know."

HF education nurse: "Start with walking in your home 5 minutes a day and add an additional 5 minutes every day. Stop if you start to feel chest discomfort or increased shortness of breath. Sit down and rest for a while then try to walk again later in the day.

Mr. S.: "I will give a try. I really want to go to my grandson's graduation."

HF education nurse: One more thing, Mr. S, Would you please keep a log of your exercise and other daily activities.

Journal writing facilitates self-analysis and reflection.[2,7] Patients were also expected to evaluate their responses to the activities performed. Journal writing requires basic writing skills and may not be suitable to patients who have limited writing ability. Alternatively, patients could use tape recorder to capture their self-evaluation activities.

WHAT ARE THE MOST APPROPRIATE METHODS TO EVALUATE HOW WELL A PATIENT HAS ACHIEVED THE REQUIRED COMPETENCIES?

Evaluation is the process of collecting and interpreting information for making judgment and providing evidence about learner achievement of learning outcome objectives. Different objectives require different evaluation methods. To ensure content validity, the evaluation tasks should not only reflect the objectives, but also reflect the instruction. Based on analysis of the learning outcome objectives and instructional activities in the context of both content knowledge and cognitive levels, the HF education nurse selected the evaluation methods listed below.

Evaluation of objective 1 required that patients understand the meaning of defined concepts. Both short-answer and multiple-choice formats are appropriate.[3] The intent is to increase the probability that understanding rather than remembering is being evaluated. For the short-answer questions, patients can be asked to explain concepts in their own words. For the multiple-choice format, patients can be asked to recognize parallel interpretations of the concepts taught. For patients with limited reading and writing skills, patient educators may read the questions and ask for verbal responses. Sample questions used for evaluation of objective 1 follow:

Use your own words to explain the meaning of congestive heart failure (CHF).

Which symptom is most likely related to worsening CHF and needs to be reported to the doctor?

   a. Headache

   b. Pale skin

   c. Sitting up to breathe at night

   d. Weight gain of 1 pound over 1 week

Evaluation of objective 2 involved tasks that required patients to analyze how component concepts relate to one another. Analysis can be evaluated with multiple-choice format. Learners are given a set of data and have to decide which information is most relevant and what action(s) to take. To construct multiple-choice items at the cognitive level of analysis, the scenario or situation presented must be novel.[13–15] Using the exact same scenario presented during instruction only yields evidence of remembering. In addition, all selection options should be plausible. Implausible selection options allow students to use the process of elimination to arrive at the correct answer. Choosing the most appropriate/relevant option from all plausible alternatives requires discriminating judgment.[13–15] An example used for evaluation of objective 2 follows:

Mrs. A. was just diagnosed with new onset of CHF. She is to see a nurse at the HF clinic for further teaching on managing her symptoms. At her most recent physician's appointment, she received the following orders: lisinopril (Zestril) 20 mg by mouth daily, furosemide (Lasix) 40 mg by mouth daily, and potassium chloride 20 mEq by mouth daily. She takes her blood pressure daily, and today's reading was 98/70. She feels very weak and short of breath. What do you think Mrs. A. should do?

   a. Take all of the medicines

   b. Take Zestril only

   c. Take Lasix only

   d. Hold all medicines and call the doctor

Sometimes it is difficult to design plausible distractors (incorrect options) for a question using a specific clinical scenario. In this case, patient educators can use common patient misconceptions or generated phrases that sound correct. Another strategy is to design homogeneous alternatives that reflect parallel content and grammatical structure so that patients must make finer distinctions among similarities.[13–15]

Evaluation of objective 3 involved judging the patients' abilities to use principles of dietary modification. In addition to knowledge, the evaluation task must measure integration of knowledge in real-world situations. Simulation allows for direct observation of learner's performance involved with making a number of decisions in a realistic environment. Shopping in a mock supermarket to plan a 2 g sodium diet was used to evaluate learning outcome for objective 3. Foods presented for the evaluation task were similar but different from the ones used for instruction.

Evaluation of objective 4 involved judging patients' behavior modification. Behavior change occurs over time. Although instruction activities for modifying patient behavior usually begin before discharge, much of actual learning occurs in the home. When opportunities for direct observation are lacking, patients' verbal or written reports may provide relevant data for evaluating compliance with medical regimen.[4] After being discharged, individual patients met with the HF education nurse weekly to review logs and determine level of achievement. The process required patients to analyze and evaluate their own performance.

HOW SHOULD THE EVIDENCE OF LEARNING BEING DOCUMENTED?

To promote interdisciplinary communication, continuity of care, and support quality improvement efforts, written documentation of all aspects of patient education is critical. To meet JCAHO standards, documentation of patient education should reflect essential information for self-care, instructional activities, evaluation methods used, and specific actual outcomes.[1] Samples of documentation for each learning objective are listed below.

Documentation for learning outcome objective 1:

Patient education on HF pathophysiology and signs/symptoms was completed using didactic presentation accompanied with graphics and printed materials. Upon completion of the session, the patient was able to explain the disease process and signs and symptoms of worsening HF in her/his own words.

Documentation for learning outcomes objective 2:

Patient education on pharmacologic therapy was completed using didactic presentation and case studies. Upon completion of the session, the patient was able to distinguish undesirable responses from expected responses to medications and determine appropriate actions from given scenarios.

Documentation for learning objective 3:

Patient education on dietary modification was completed using simulated grocery shopping. Upon completion of the instructional activity, the patient was able to choose low-sodium foods from the available items and correctly calculate the total amount of sodium content from the foods chosen.

Documentation for learning objective 4:

Patient education on activity/exercise modification was completed before discharge using 1:1 reflective discussion of strategies for improving activity/exercise tolerance in relation to personal goals. Self-reported logs were reviewed during the meeting held at HF clinic 1 week after being discharged. The patient stated in the logs: "I want to be able to attend my grandson's graduation." "I walked everyday for 5 minutes without stopping. I was more short of breath on the first day. I felt much better by day #3."

RELATING EVALUATION DATA TO TEACHING–LEARNING PROCESS

Evaluation measures the degree to which learning outcome objectives have been met. Evaluation results are used to inform patients of areas for improvement. In addition, educators should use evaluation data to gain insight into the effectiveness of each element of the teaching–learning process. If the patient was not able to achieve the intended learning, the HF education nurse would reexamine the process for congruence among learning outcome objectives, instruction, and evaluation methods. The HF education nurse would also reassess: whether the learning outcome objectives were realistic to the patient's situation, whether the instructional activities reflected the patient's background, and whether the evaluation methods were appropriate to elicit the outcome behaviors.

SUMMARY

To ensure that patients attain the required abilities for self-management, patient education needs to be competency-based. The main focus of competency-based education is on the outcomes; instructional activities and evaluation methods must be carefully aligned with the intended learning outcome objectives.[2,3] Incongruence among these elements may result in ineffective patient education.[3]

When developing and applying a competency-based patient education lesson/ program, each nurse must answer the following questions:

What are the essential competencies for patient self-management of health?
What teaching methods will yield the intended learning?
What are the most appropriate methods to evaluate how well a patient has achieved the competencies?
How should the evidence of learning be documented?[2,3]

No 1 teaching method is suitable for every outcome objective and patient, and no 1 evaluation format provides exhaustive data for judging patient performance. It is important to use multiple instruction and evaluation strategies based on the nature of each patient's ability to learn.

In this article, the authors described how they used these questions and principles as guides to achieve congruence among intended learning, instruction, and evaluation of a patient education program, Managing Heart Failure, at a local hospital.

REFERENCES

1. The Joint Commission of Accreditation of Hospital Organizations. CAMH Comprehensive accreditation manual for hospitals. Oak brook Terrace (IL): Joint Commission; 2006.
2. Anema M, McCoy J. Competence-based nursing education. New York: Springer Publishing Company; 2010.
3. Anderson LW, Krathwohl DR, Airasian PW, et al. A taxonomy for learning, teaching, and assessing: a revision of Bloom's Taxonomy of educational objectives. New York: Addison Wesley Longman; 2001.
4. Jessup M, Abraham W, Casey D, et al. Focused update: ACCF/AHA practice guidelines for the diagnosis and management of heart failure in adults. Circulation 2009;119:1977–2016.
5. Rankin S, Stallings K, London F. Patient education in health and illness. 5th edition. Philadelphia: Lippincott Williams & Wilkins; 2005.
6. Su WM, Osisek PJ, Starnes B. Applying the revised Bloom's Taxonomy to a medical–surgical nursing lesson. Nurse Educ 2004;29(3):116–20.
7. Benner P, Sutphen M, Leonard V, et al. Educating nurses: a call for radical transformation. Standford (CA): Jossey-Bass; 2010.
8. Suter PM, Suter WN. Timeless principles of learning: a solid foundation for enhancing chronic disease self-management. Home Healthc Nurse 2008;26(2): 83–8.
9. Gaberson KB, Oermann MH. Clinical teaching strategies in nursing. 3rd edition. New York: Spring Publishing Company; 2010.

10. Redman BK. The practice of patient education: a case study approach. 3rd edition. St Louis (MO): Mosby; 2007.
11. Alfaro-Lefvre R. Critical thinking and clinical judgment in nursing. 4th edition. St Louis (MO): Saunders; 2009.
12. Pintrich PR. The role of metacognitive knowledge in learning, teaching, and assessing. Theory Pract 2002;41(4):219–25.
13. Morrison S, Nibert A, Flick J. Critical thinking and test item writing. 2nd edition. Houston (TX): Health Education System; 2006.
14. Oermann MH, Gaberson KB. Evaluation and testing in nursing education. 3rd edition. New York: Springer Publishing Company; 2009.
15. Su WM, Osisek PJ, Montgomery C, et al. Designing multiple-choice test items at higher cognitive levels. Nurse Educ 2009;34(5):223–7.

Creating Educational Objectives for Patient Education Using the New Bloom's Taxonomy

Stephen D. Krau, PhD, RN, CNE

KEYWORDS

- Patient education • Educational objectives
- Bloom's Taxonomy

Inherent in a patient-nurse interaction is some form of teaching. Whenever the nurse encounters a patient or a patient's family, there is a transfer of some information that either implicitly or explicitly is expected to be incorporated into the patient's overall outcome. Much teaching is informal and is not well documented, and the level to which the patient understands is often not well evaluated and poorly documented. The creation of objectives for patient education helps to guide the instructional process by coordinating the plan for teaching and patient learning. In addition, objectives provide a basis for the evaluation as to what extent learning has occurred, as objectives provide a standard by which to measure patient behavior. Moreover, objectives focus the educational encounter or session toward patient learning and away from the educator or the process itself. Many nurses are familiar with educational objectives as a result of their own educational experiences in a nursing program or continuing education classes. Creating educational objectives that are patient focused is different from using objectives as a learner. To create meaningful and patient-oriented objectives, the nurse has many issues to consider.

Developing learning objectives that are patient focused directs the focus of the encounter toward specific learning as opposed to transmitting volume of information that may not be completely useful to the patient. The creation of patient-centered learning objectives takes the focus of the encounter away from the nurse and directs it toward the patient. In addition, when there are multiple persons involved in the educational process, objectives help provide continuity of focus. To be effective, the objectives must consider the needs and the learning style of the patient, and serve as a fundamental guide that teaching contributes to an outcome rather than to an end in itself.[1]

The author has nothing to disclose.
Vanderbilt University Medical Center, School of Nursing, 461 21st Avenue, South Nashville, TN 37240, USA
E-mail address: steve.krau@vanderbilt.edu

doi:10.1016/j.cnur.2011.05.002
0029-6465/11/$ – see front matter © 2011 Elsevier Inc. All rights reserved.
nursing.theclinics.com

OBJECTIVES VERSUS OUTCOMES

To create and evaluate objectives, a clear understanding of what constitutes an "objective" and how this differs from an "outcome" is essential. Nurses traditionally have been taught to begin educational encounters with an explanation of objectives for that educational encounter. Objectives provide a clear understanding of the purpose of the session and help to illuminate the expectations of the person teaching that session.[2] To that end, there is some demonstrable change that occurs in the learner that can be evaluated by the teacher as evidence that learning has occurred. As stated by Rankin and Stallings in 2001, "Objectives describe behaviors that the learner will perform to meet a goal."[3(p240)]

Changes in health care have led to an emphasis on outcomes. For this reason it is important to discuss educational outcomes as they relate to learning outcomes and not necessarily overall patient outcomes. The nomenclature can, and does, get confusing as teaching and learning is directed toward learning objectives and educational outcomes which, it is hoped, will contribute to the overall patient outcome. Within the realm of education, the term "outcome" has infiltrated nursing education and is frequently used synonymously with the term "objective."[4,5] Educational literature has often mentioned outcomes in an attempt to redirect the learning/teaching process toward the learner as opposed to the teacher and learner, or the process itself. A review of the standard definitions of the words "objective" and "outcome" reveals significant differences in the concepts.[2] An objective considers the process and the goal, and is inherently teacher and student focused. An outcome considers the end product or goal, and inherently focuses on the student, as learning is the goal for the student.

Beyond the semantics, educational outcomes and objectives might be considered with regard to their levels of measurement. For example, the objective for a teaching encounter with newly diagnosed diabetes might be related to explaining the differences between regular and NPH insulin. The process focuses on the student's ability to articulate information about regular insulin and NPH insulin, and to draw conclusions for comparison. The objective organizes the interaction, provides clear focus for the discussion, and provides criteria for evaluation. The scope is limited to information about the two different types of insulin. Information about how to administer insulin and the physiologic effect of insulin on the disease process would be subsumed in another objective or group of objectives. An outcome related to the end product or goal of patient teaching would focus on the patient's overall ability to medically manage and control the diabetic disease process. The educational outcome is focused on a synthesis of knowledge, skills, and motivation, with an end result being safe administration of medication based on glucose levels. An overall patient outcome would consider the totality of the patient's ability to manage a disease process or maintain an optimal level of health. A patient outcome is broader in scope and would be measured by such standards as the number of hospital admissions for complications related to diabetes, or number of office visits indicating that glucose levels are being maintained within normal ranges. Educational objectives and educational outcomes might have contributed to the overall outcome, but the overall outcome is broader in scope.

There is as much discussion about the merits of educational outcomes over educational objectives as there is about the differences. There are those who maintain that educational outcomes reflect the students' performance in relation to educational objectives.[4] As stated by Prideaux, "It is difficult to explain the difference between a significant and worthwhile objective and a well-written and well-defined outcome."[6(p169)] Educational outcomes and objectives still focus on the learner, the behavior, and the content, and provide means to evaluate the efficiency of the inter-action. Limits related to scope, and overall expectations of the client, are essential to viable objectives and outcomes. Differences in nursing education and patient educa-tion are also considered here, as there is much discussion about learning outcomes for students as adult learners. In these situations, nurses want students to be crea-tive, to solve problems, and to be less restrictive. Outcomes are considered slightly less restrictive in the learning environment and a move toward education processes that are more liberating.[7] When considering patient education, much of what is taught is based on evidence, protocols, and standards. Whereas creativity might be a component, there is usually foundational information that must be mastered before moving toward creative thinking and more creative outcomes. In some cases, foundational information leads to creative solutions and creative behaviors; however, there is a hierarchy of the level of information and expected behaviors. Many of these levels and the relationships among these levels are reflected in what is typically called a "taxonomy."

TAXONOMIES OF OBJECTIVES

Objectives are typically written to reflect 1 of 3 domains, which include cognitive, affective, and psychomotor. The cognitive domain focuses on knowledge and intellec-tual skills. Objectives in this domain would focus on the acquisition of information and specific facts related to the management or control of a disease process, or to promote health. **Table 1** demonstrates the levels of this domain as presented by the Revised Bloom's Taxonomy.

The affective domain focuses on the development of values, attitudes, and beliefs. The taxonomy developed by Krathwohl, Bloom, and Masia includes 5 levels that prog-ress from the basic awareness of a value to the internalization of a value. The internal-ization of a value forms a basis for behavior.[8] The value is reflected in decision making, and inherently there is a cognitive base for the development of a system of values. It is important to consider this domain in patient teaching, as it will help identify to what extent there is a common value between the health care professional and the patient. For example, if management of a disease process enables independence, the value of independence might be different for the patient and the nurse educator. The meaning of independence may also vary and carry other values. Independence may entail a better economic outcome with better management of a disease process, resulting in fewer or shorter hospital stays or less time missed from employment. Or, if the value is related to family, less time away from the hospital would provide the patient with more time with the family, which may be the motivation for the patient to learn what is being taught. Many objectives and goals based on this domain are driven by the consensus of the system within which the patient receives care. As such, the accom-plishment or degree to which objectives based on the affective domain are attained can only be determined over time.

There are several interpretations and presentations of the psychomotor domain. The original committee that formulated Bloom's Taxonomy did not produce a compilation of the psychomotor domain. There have been others who have done so in more recent years, which explains why this domain varies in detail through different interpretations. The most popular referenced versions of this domain include those created R.H. Dave,[9] E.J. Simpson,[10] and A.J. Harrow.[11] The domains are quite different, but underlying each level is the tenet that the cognitive domain is present. A presentation of the 3 domains, with the psychomotor domain as interpreted by Dave,[9] is given in **Fig. 1**.

Table 1
The cognitive processing dimension of the Revised Bloom's Taxonomy

Dimension	Examples of the Cognitive Processes Involved	Patient Objective Related to the Dimension
Remember To what extent can the patient recall or remember the information?	Define, Duplicate, List, Memorize, Recall, Recognize, Record, Repeat, Reproduce, State	The patient will define left-sided heart failure The patient will memorize the names of the medications used to manage diabetes
Understand To what extent can the patient explain the ideas or concepts?	Classify, Describe, Discuss, Explain, Exemplify, Identify, Interpret, Locate, Paraphrase, Recognize, Report, Select, Translate	The patient will explain the effect of calcium channel blockers on the cardiovascular system The patient will describe the mechanism of hyperglycemia
Apply To what extent can the patient use the information in a new way?	Choose, Demonstrate, Dramatize, Employ, Execute, Illustrate, Implement, Operate, Schedule, Sketch, Solve, Use, Write	The patient will choose from a list foods that are low in fats and carbohydrates
Analyze To what extent can the patient distinguish between or among different parts?	Appraise, Attribute, Compare, Contrast, Criticize, Differentiate, Discriminate, Distinguish, Examine, Experiment, Question, Organize, Test	The patient will differentiate between short-acting and long-acting insulin
Evaluate To what extent can the student justify a stand or position?	Appraise, Argue, Check, Critique, Defend, Judge, Select, Support, Value, Evaluate	The patient will critique the foods in a meal for their impact on blood glucose levels
Create To what extent can the patient create a new product or point of view?	Assemble, Build, Construct, Create, Design, Develop, Formulate, Generate, Plan, Produce	The patient will develop a month plan of meals that meet with his or her therapeutic regimen

A valuable framework for the development of student objectives in an educational setting and provision of guidance for patient-centered learning objectives is *Bloom's Taxonomy of Educational Objectives*. Published in 1956, this volume has been a mainstay for the organization of objectives, levels of cognition, and psychomotor and affective domains of education. Newer knowledge as to how humans learn as well as how to assess learning has been slow to infiltrate academic environments and even slower to permeate other settings, including the health care milieu. To understand the progression of the taxonomy and the potential impact on current patient education, it is helpful to examine its historical development and to appraise its value in relation to the formulation of patient-centered outcomes.

HISTORICAL PERSPECTIVE

The value of Bloom's work is unquestionable. Although named after Benjamin Bloom, the original taxonomy was the work of many persons who were tasked to help manage the tremendous influx of military veterans into the academic system following World

Cognitive Domain

Concerned with intellectual objectives. Considered the central point of most tests that are developed, as it deals with the development of intellectual ability. Tools to assess a patient's knowledge of a disease process, or how to manage and illness and illness would be subsumed in this domain.

Evaluation

This includes the ability to employ criteria or standards to make judgments with regard to the value of ideas, solutions, and methods. Evaluation requires all other levels of cognition.

Synthesis

The ability to combine elements to create a new idea, object, or procedure. This level requires creativity on the part of the patient as something is created that was not previously there.

Analysis

The ability to breakdown material or content into its components or parts so its organizational structure is comprehended. This requires a patient to disassemble parts, examine the relationships among the parts, recognize effects, and comprehend the meaning of the information.

Application

The ability to use learned material in new and concrete situations. Here, the patient is to use abstractions to apply concepts, laws, methods, phenomena, principles, procedures, rules and theories to solve problems.

Comprehension

This encompasses the notion that the patient is able to grasp the overall meaning of what is being taught. This is inherent in the ability to translate information from one form to another. This is often evaluated by asking the patient to express in "their own words" what has just been explained.

Knowledge

This is essentially the ability of the patient to recall previously learned material. As the lowest level of the taxonomy, it involves simple recall of a fact, concept, theory or principle. At this level the patient is expected to remember information exactly as it was presented.

Affective Domain

Objectives in this domain involve interests, attitudes and values. As they relate to patient education, characteristics impact on how the patient will respond to teaching, perceives the meaning of the disease process, and how impacts issues of importance to the patient. This includes the manner in which patients deal with things emotionally.

Characterizing by Value

Inherently, this level is achieved when the patient's value system "controls" his or her behavior. The behavior becomes the characteristic of the patient and is pervasive, consistent and predictable.

Organizing or Conceptualizing

This is concerned with prioritization based on values. Identifying contrasting and different values and reconciling them creating a unique system of values. The emphasis is on comparing values, and synthesizing values. Essentially, at the level, the patient reconciles internal conflicts as they develop a value system toward what is being taught.

Valuing

This level centers on the worth that a patient attaches to a particular object or behavior. This can range from acceptance to a strong sense of commitment. This is based primarily on the extent to which the patient has internalized a set of specific values. Clues to these values are often identifiable in the patient's overt behavior.

Responding

This involves active participation on the part of the learner. The student not only attends to a stimulus, but also reacts in some manner. Related to this level, learning objectives may center around compliance in responding, willingness to respond, or degree of satisfaction in responding or motivation.

Receiving

This level is concerned with the patient's awareness, willingness to listen, and selected attention. Without this level, no learning can occur.

Psychomotor Domain

RH Dave's Version

These involve objectives that are motor skill oriented and concerned with movements that require coordination, and control. Psychomotor skills inherently contain a cognitive aspect, involving understanding related to the skill, and affective aspect that is concerned with a patient's values and attitudes while performing a skill.

Naturalization

This encompasses an instinctive and effortless unconscious mastery of and activity and skills related to that activity. Essentially, the response is automatic and can be completed without deliberation.

Articulation

At this level, the patient is able to adapt and integrate expertise to satisfy a new task or a previous task within a new context. In this case, the patient would be expected to relate and combine associated activities to develop methods to address variant and novel situations.

Precision

This level is focused on the patient's ability to execute a skill reliably, and independent of help. The activity is executed quickly, smoothly, and with accuracy with minimal energy expenditure. The skill is performed without hesitation, with fewer errors.

Manipulation

This occurs when the patient can reproduce an activity from a previous instruction or from memory. This would occur when a patient can perform a task from memory and not from immediate prior instruction. The skill can be performed with confidence and some proficiency.

Imitation

This level is characterized by a patient copying an action of another, or observing and replicating what is observed. This is essentially what is occurring when a "return demonstration" is expected. This is done by the patient under close supervision of the nurse. When presenting a new skill to the patient, the nurse should present the knowledge context first, then the skill should be broken down into very basic parts for the patient. During the return demonstration, the nurse should not quiz the patient about theoretical matters, or interrupt the patient's train of thought.

Fig. 1. Comparison of the 3 domains of Bloom's Taxonomy.

War II.[12] After World War II many veterans were eligible for GI (Government Issue) benefits, which facilitated the admission of many veterans into the academic environment as students. These veterans had considerable "life experience," which was recognized by the academicians and acknowledged by the Department of Defense (DOD). These factors resulted in the emergence of the practice of granting college credit by examination. To organize and maintain rigor and credibility in the examination process, the Taxonomy of Education emerged.[12]

Persons involved in the endeavor to create, administer, and evaluate these tests were referred to as "Examiners."[12] As Examiners were primarily in the field of psychology, the inaugural meeting of the collective Examiners occurred at the annual meeting of the American Psychological Association in 1948. There were ongoing meetings with the purpose of identifying, classifying, and structuring intellectual content for the awarding of credit by examination. Borrowing from the scheme proposed by natural scientists to organize plants and animals from simple to complex, the Examiners identified the Kingdoms of Life Taxonomy as a format from which to create a hierarchy for a framework for creating examinations on a variety of topics.[13] The group decided that this design would provide an effective system for categorizing levels of knowledge for their tests.[14]

The Examiners concurred that a classification system embodied an appropriate foundation to measure student knowledge and understanding. Through a system for identifying criteria, developing test items, and evaluating students, it was held that educators would be able to make better comparisons and study educational programming.[12] By 1956, the efforts resulted in *Bloom's Taxonomy of Educational Objectives*, named by default because Benjamin Bloom was alphabetically the first name in the list of authors. This seminal work has been a cornerstone for curriculum design and development, for test construction, and for student evaluation for more than half a century. The original authors have maintained that the work is continually in progress, and that it is neither finished nor final.[14]

The original taxonomy has been used extensively by educators in allied health fields and nursing to structure lesson plans and evaluate student learning. Bloom's Taxonomy is currently referred to as the Revised Bloom's Taxonomy (RT) following its update in 2001. The hierarchy consists of 3 different domains of learning, which include cognitive, affective, and psychomotor, as identified in **Fig. 1**. Within the taxonomic levels, higher learning is contingent on initial learning at the lower levels. The revised taxonomy has already been used in patient education as a framework to teach diagnostic reasoning to clients with myocardial infarctions. Their use of the taxonomy demonstrated congruence among learning and the evaluation of that learning.[15]

More recently, Marzano and Kendall[16] have developed a new taxonomy for educational objectives that not only considers how humans make a decision to initiate a new task but also elucidates how information is processed once that decision has been made. Their model incorporates the ideas of 3 mental systems in this process, which include the self-system, the metacognitive system, and the cognitive system. Their work incorporates the newest information on human cognition and extends the work of others. It adds dimensions to the practical applicability of taxonomic levels in the development of curriculum.

BLOOM'S ORIGINAL TAXONOMY

The value of Bloom's Original Taxonomy (OT) to education and the formulation of educational objectives is impressive. The taxonomy includes 6 major categories in the cognitive domain, namely Knowledge, Comprehension, Application, Analysis, Synthesis, and Evaluation.[17] The categories are ordered from simple to complex in a linear manner from concrete to abstract. It is assumed that this taxonomy represented a cumulative hierarchy, which means that movement to the next-level category is predicated on mastery of the previous-level category.

The purpose of the taxonomy was to provide a system by which to classify educational goals. One of the most frequent uses for the OT has been to classify curricular objectives and develop test items to demonstrate the span of the objectives across the spectrum of the 6 categories.[18,19] Bloom identified the OT as more than a measurement tool, in that the tool had a multifaceted utility. The OT provided: (1) a common language about learning goals to facilitate communication across persons and subject matter; (2) a basis for providing meaning to broad educational goals at multiple local, state, and national levels; (3) a means of congruence for the objectives of a course, or educational activities, and appraisal in a unit, course, or curriculum; and (4) a panorama of educational possibilities against which the breadth and depth of any particular educational course or curriculum could be considered.[19(p12)]

Reasons the OT Warranted Revision

There are several weaknesses and limitations of the OT that have been identified over the years. A major weakness relates to an assumption that cognitive processes evolve and are ordered on a single dimension of such from simple to complex.[20] As the OT is a hierarchy that is cumulative, there is an inherent assumption that the categories do not overlap or interchange. This standard has reported issues with the frequent inversion of various objectives and tasks. That is to say, certain demands for knowledge might actually be more complex than certain demands for Analysis or Evaluation.[18] In addition, Evaluation is not inherently more complex than Synthesis, because Synthesis involves Evaluation.[21(p65)]

BLOOM'S REVISED TAXONOMY

Due to more recent thought in learning and teaching, with an emphasis on students or patients being more knowledgable and more responsible for their own learning, it was necessary that new learning paradigms be incorporated into the taxonomy. To address the limitations of the OT and to remain current with the shifts in educational thought, a group of cognitive psychologists, curriculum and instructional researchers, and testing and assessment specialists revised the OT.[14]

At first glance the differences between the OT and RT might not be evident. Closer examination indicates that a change from the OT to the RT is associated with the verbiage of moving from nouns to verbs in different levels of the taxonomy. For the most part, the top 2 levels are essentially unchanged. In addition, in the knowledge category there are now 2 dimensions. Whereas formally the subcategories under the knowledge category contained both noun and verb, the presentation was unidimensional in identifying that knowledge was dual in nature, unlike the other categories. In the RT these two aspects are not mutually exclusive or dualistic, but rather allow the noun to provide the basis for the knowledge dimension and the verb to form the basis for a dimension of cognitive process, making the category 2-dimensional. Thus, statements of objectives in the RT will consist of a subject matter in the form of a noun or noun phrase, and a description of what is to be done with that content as a verb or verb phrase. The verb phrase then becomes the cognitive process that is involved in the completion of the objective.

Changes in the Knowledge Dimension

Advances in educational and cognitive psychology have brought new awareness to human thinking processes, evoking the need for a new taxonomy that incorporates this new information. Thus there is an additional category in the Knowledge category of the RT that is not present in the OT. The Knowledge category was revised to reflect the distinctions of cognitive psychology. Many educators today realize that recall and memorization of facts is not particularly important because so much information is available through the Internet. However, with patients this may not be the case, as physiologic events can impede the patient's ability to access the information, and not all patients have immediate access. This nuance in patient education does not correlate with information access commonly seen in a school or academic setting. Hence, the value of recall and memorization when it leads to an action is an important consideration in the management of many disease processes. The categories in the RT related to knowledge were reorganized, and another category was added.

Changes in the Cognitive Process Dimension

Both taxonomies have 6 categories but are not the same. Three categories were renamed, and the order of 2 of the categories was changed. The revised categories were changed from noun form to verb form to better fit the syntax for formulating objectives. The revised names were changed to Remembering, Understanding, and Creating. Differences between the OT and the RT are demonstrated in **Fig. 2**.

Factual knowledge is essentially the basic elements that a patient must know to be acquainted with a disease, or potential health care deviation, or to solve problems associated with these. *Conceptual knowledge* consists of the interrelationships among basic elements within a larger context or structure that enable them to function in concert. *Procedural knowledge* consists of methods of completing a task, methods of inquiry, and criteria for using skills, algorithms, techniques, and methods. This process typically involves a set of steps, or a sequence or series of steps to follow. *Metacognitive knowledge* is the new dimension that was added. This aspect consists of the awareness and knowledge of one's own cognition as well as the knowledge of cognition in general.[22] The metacognitive component conveys a paradigm shift in education from the OT to the RT toward making students more aware and responsible for their learning. It embodies the idea that students or patients who know about different strategies of learning, thinking, and solving problems will most likely use them. Patients who are aware of their personal strengths or limitations can adjust learning and contribute to learning strategies more conducive to their learning needs. Metacognition is also related to the transfer of learning, or the ability to use knowledge

New Bloom's Taxonomy		Old Bloom's Taxonomy
Cognitive Process	**Knowledge Dimension**	
Creating	Metacognitive	Evaluation
Evaluating	Metacognitive	Synthesis
Analyzing	Metacognitive	Analysis
Applying	Procedural	Application
Understanding	Conceptual	Comprehension
Remembering	Factual	Knowledge

Fig. 2. The differences between the new Bloom's Taxonomy and the old Bloom's Taxonomy.

acquired in one setting or situation in another.[23] This concept is congruent to the trends in health care whereby today patients are going home with higher acuity than 40 years ago, and have considerably shorter hospital stays. The management of disease processes or health promotion is much more patient centered and relies heavily on the patient's awareness and knowledge. One method that promotes the metacognitive process in patient education is to have patients create logs for variant physiologic measurements over time, or to keep a journal and write reflections.

The major contribution that the RT can make to the educational process is inherent in the manner in which nurses involved in patient education will think about the teaching session and manner of instruction. The blending of cognitive processes and the knowledge dimension can enhance instructional planning and evaluation. When determining the best method to evaluate learning, educators will consider the myriad of learning activities for the interaction. A strategy proposed by Packard[12] to help educators formulate a conceptualization of the RT is to use the metaphor of a cooking recipe. In a standard recipe, the format usually consists of a list of ingredients followed by directions as to how to combine and cook the ingredients for the desired outcome. In essence, the list of ingredients is *factual knowledge*, while the directions for the method of preparing the recipe are a series of steps, or *procedural knowledge*. *Conceptual knowledge* enters as the person preparing the recipe makes appropriate substitutions. *Metacognitive knowledge* allows the learner to make appropriate and strategic modifications in the procedure, and would form the basis of knowing which recipes to avoid at variant altitudes and variant humidity. *Metacognition* would also be observed when the person preparing the meal can combine ingredients on hand to complete a meal without referring to a recipe or menu, or when the person can prepare a meal with foods readily at hand. This metacognitive knowledge, in addition to factual and procedural knowledge, is typically used when preparing recipes from foods that have been purchased for that set recipe.[12]

This metaphor in a patient situation could be related to teaching a patient about diet management. Early on, the patient would need basic information about proteins, carbohydrates, and fats and how they work, and their impact on blood glucose levels. This information would constitute knowledge that is factual. Then the patient would most likely learn how to plan and create meals that fall within therapeutic parameters for himself or herself. At this point the patient might rely on readings, handouts, calorie and constituent counters, and a set of steps or recipes to prepare a meal; this would constitute procedural knowledge. An example of metacognitive knowledge related to this scenario would be the patient's ability to dine in a restaurant, and make appropriate choices and adaptations to a meal outside the patient's own kitchen, but remaining within the therapeutic parameters of the patient's dietary restrictions. A nurse educator would hardly expect a patient to be able to make restaurant adaptations without first understanding the principle of *what* is to be adapted.

Writing Objectives Using the RT

One way to determine the extent to which a patient is knowledgable is to observe the patient's behavior. The RT presents the knowledge domain as a hierarchy of verbs, whereas the early taxonomy expressed the levels in nouns. Verbs are an indicator of behavior, making the RT more congruent to behaviors expected as the result of an educational encounter. For example, a general learning objective requires that a newly diagnosed patient perform procedures to control the disease process. The value of controlling the disease process is unquestionable, but the behaviors inferred in this goal are not clear. The objective is really more of an overall outcome that can be measured by the specific behaviors that contribute to the safe management of the disease process. In order for the outcome to become the basis for instruction and evaluation, the expected behaviors should be presented as objectives. **Table 2** presents a generic example whereby the management of the disease is contingent on considerations related to medications, diet, and exercise.

The same example could be applied to any variety of health care issues, regarding for example a patient who has been diagnosed with diabetes, a patient who has recently been diagnosed with cardiovascular disease, or a patient who is being treated for obesity or eating disorders. For different disease processes there may be other factors to consider, but for purposes of example, perusal of how the objectives are behaviorally written help the nurse evaluate the extent to which the patient has mastered the objective.

Depending on the disease process or health requirements, the outcomes will vary. The presented objectives could be refined to reflect specific issues related to the disease process, or individualized based on the patient's needs. For example, in selecting equipment for exercise, a diabetic patient would need to consider appropriate foot care. When considering food, a diabetic would need to consider the amount of carbohydrates, whereas a major consideration for a cardiovascular patient would be the amount of salt in the diet. This area is where nursing knowledge is integral to the educational process, and where resources are accessed to develop more focused objectives for that particular patient. **Table 2** shows how specific objectives contribute to the overall outcome.

CREATING INSTRUCTIONAL OBJECTIVES FOR PATIENT EDUCATION

The nurse who is educating the patient will consider what is to be taught, and what level of knowledge, affect, or psychomotor skill is appropriate for the creating an objective. There are several important considerations to consider when creating educational objectives. As the focus of the interaction will be the behaviors of the patient, the objectives are to be written in terms of patient behaviors, not the behaviors of the nurse or other health care provider. The purpose of the objectives is to focus the instruction on the behaviors that will be observed and measured in the patient.[24] To this end, it would be appropriate to begin each objective, or a list of objectives, with the phase: "The patient will...."

The objectives must be measurable. Focusing on specific behaviors allows the patient to demonstrate what they have learned, while the nurse observes and evaluates the behavior as evidence that learning has occurred. A common error in writing

Table 2
A general outcome with learning objectives

	Medication	Diet	Exercise
1. Outcome: The patient will safely manage and control the diabetic disease process			
1.1 Discuss rationale	X	X	X
1.2 Identifies impact	X	X	X
1.3 Explains procedures as related	X	X	X
1.4 Selects equipment or appropriate foods	X	X	X
1.5 Completes procedure	X	X	X
1.6 Interprets response	X	X	X
1.7 Addresses response	X	X	X

objectives is the use of words such as "understand," "think," or "know," which are not observable behaviors and cannot be measured. The patient may "verbalize" that he or she "understands" something, but that does not provide evidence that what is being taught is actually understood. Behavioral measurements allow the nurse to see to what extent learning has occurred. The objectives should identify opportunities for the nurse to discern the level of understanding through observable and measurable behaviors.

These behaviors can be the result of a skill that is demonstrated, or the score on a written quiz or test of the material. Demonstrating a skill is very different from describing a skill or listing the steps of a skill. For example, consider the common skill of riding a bicycle. One may know about the physical properties of balance, movement, and speed as they relate to riding a bicycle. However, understanding these concepts as they relate to this skill does not mean that one can actually *perform* the skill. There also other attributes that warrant consideration in the development of effective patient objectives. Some of these attributes suggested by Huba and Freed[25] are presented in **Table 3**.

The specific content, skill, or behavior that is to be demonstrated must be included in each instructional objective. The behavior and the manner in which the patient is to demonstrate the behavior must be unmistakable.[26] Stating the objective first and then listing a representative sample of performance standards clarifies for the learner what is acceptable to the teacher as evidence of attaining the objective. The degree of specificity is contingent on the level of interaction and overall level of the student. For example, a specific instructional objective might be "Within 10 minutes of instruction (10 minutes is a condition), the patient (learner) will obtain (behavior) a blood glucose level and determine the amount of regular insulin to be administered (criterion)." Often objectives that are this specific can lead the patient to focus on elements that are not as essential. In this example, the condition is not as important as the behavior or the criterion; however, this can become the patient's focus. So rather than having a complex objective, the alternative is to have more objectives to encompass what is expected. In this example, the patient is expected to perform a glucose level, and to choose the correct amount of insulin based on that level; these could easily be two objectives that are clear and lend themselves to be evaluated separately. The condition, in this case, might not be as important as it could be in other scenarios.

USING INSTRUCTIONAL OBJECTIVES FOR PATIENT EDUCATION

Once objectives that correlate to the patient's diagnosis and learning needs are formulated, it is important to communicate these to the patient. This contact directs the teaching interaction, keeps the focus on the patient's learning needs, and keeps the learning session from redirection toward broad topics and unrestricted information. The emphasis in the RT is on educational objectives, which help educators delineate and communicate what they intend students to learn as the result of the teaching interaction.

The objectives provide a plan for selecting the appropriate teaching approaches, creating learning activities and indicating how the result will be evaluated. Some objectives may designate learning outcomes in all 3 domains. It is important for the nurse to identify this occurrence so that evaluation strategies can be implemented to determine to what extent the objective has been met. Evaluation of the objective can be measured through a variety of approaches, depending on the level of knowledge, affect, or psychomotor skill. Variant evaluation strategies can include performance checklists, performance rubrics, written assignments, multiple-choice

Table 3
Criteria for effective objectives for patient education

Criterion	Explanation
Complete	An objective should be included for each important aspect of the teaching session. If the overall result is to be an educational outcome, each element of the outcome should have an objective that is evidence based, and part of a protocol that is based on best practices. All domains should be considered and should focus on higher learning as well as basic learning
Appropriate	In order for the objectives to be relevant, they must be congruent to the current evidence, and best practices protocols. Based on the learning style and medical and nursing needs of the patient, the objectives should be consistent with standards of practice
Sound	Sound objectives are compatible with the principles of teaching and learning. They must be appropriate to the experience level of the patient, must be in a language understood by the patient, and be appropriate for the developmental level of the patient. Objectives should reflect that what is being taught is permanent and should have meaning for the patient. Objectives that are not meaningful can be met during the teaching session but are usually soon forgotten
Feasible	Clearly defined and attainable objectives are more valuable than a long list of unattainable objectives. Objectives must be realistic and attainable in terms of patient ability, available time, and resources. If the patient does not have resources to achieve the objective, the objective becomes meaningless
Relevant	Objectives that are relevant can help decrease the trivia in the educational experience by focusing the interaction on what is important for the patient to manage the disease process or promote wellness. Not all patients need or want to know everything about their disease processes. They do need to know how to manage their disease, but advanced pathophysiology, while interesting to the nurse, may not always serve the best interest of the patient
Open-ended	Objectives should be clear enough to define patient behavior. They should provide direction without limiting the overall learning experience. Although this is not always desirable at lower taxonomic levels, flexibility is achieved with more open-ended objectives. Patients may adapt ideas and concepts in a manner that better reflects their values and lifestyles, but still fall within the parameters of best evidence and best practices
Delineate patient behavior	Each objective should identify the patient behavior that signifies and defines the achievement of that objective. When written in terms of patient behavior that describes learning, the objectives clarify the instructional intent and provide a basis for teaching methods, learning activities, and evaluation strategies
Shared with the patient	Although this might seem obvious, it is essential. If the objectives are well communicated to the patient, the patient realizes that the objectives are important. This supports the patient as being an active learner, and helps the patient understand and identify his or her own strengths and weaknesses in the overall process. It encourages patients to be agents and advocates in their self-care

Data from Huba ME, Freed JE. Learning-centered assessment on college campuses: shifting the focus from teaching to learning. Boston: Allyn and Bacon; 2000. p. 62.

evaluation tools, and even other written assignments such as logs or data recording. The important point is that activities should be considered for each of the objectives, and that a form of evaluation is inherent in each objective. This approach assures that every teaching encounter, activity, and procedure that is taught has a readily identifiable purpose.

SUMMARY

Instructional objectives provide a foundation for the nurse-patient teaching interaction. Objectives provide the initial step in establishing the validity of instructional methods and a means for evaluating patient behavior. The RT clarifies objectives and enables better communication with patients regarding the intended outcomes resulting from instruction. A standard format of educational objectives facilitates the nurse-patient teaching interaction, focusing the interaction on patient behavior, and provides a basis for effective evaluation of outcomes. Objectives that are written with reference to the RT take into consideration not only the behavior of the patient but also the level of cognition that is employed by the patient to achieve those objectives. As a tool for education, the objectives must be clear and have appropriate meaning for the patient. This situation can only be assured through the dynamic relationship in which nurse educators at the bedside or in classrooms engage with their patients. To be effective, the interaction must not only be communicated clearly but should also incorporate dimensions of the other domains, as the nurse discerns the meaning of the illness and the impact of the therapeutic regimen on the values and resources of the patient.

Using the two dimensions of the RT is a worthwhile complement to therapeutic patient education. Objectives based on this taxonomy lead to a patient-centered human approach, which encourages patients to be agents in their own treatment, to improve their overall quality of life, and to reduce potential complications—in essence, to contribute to the overall patient outcome that transcends the educational objective or educational outcome. As this is a fundamental purpose for nursing, it is important that all nurses, regardless of where they encounter their patients, invest the effort to learn to create sound instructional objectives and link those to the overall patient outcome. Well-written objectives will provide a means for appropriate patient evaluation, and will lead to more effective teaching interaction and documentation of learner behavior.

REFERENCES

1. MacDonald M. Developing instructional objectives. In: The nurse educator's guide to assessing learning outcomes. Sudbury (MA): Jones and Bartlett; 2007. p. 27–48.
2. Wittmann-Price RA, Fasolka BJ. Objectives and outcomes: the fundamental differences. Nurs Educ Perspect 2010;31(4):233–6.
3. Rankin S, Stallings K. Patient education: principles and practice. Philadelphia: Lippincott; 2001.
4. Morin K. Faculty questions and answers. J Nurs Educ 2007;46(6):250–1.
5. Partusch M. Assessment and evaluation strategies. In: Moyer B, Wittmann-Price RA, editors. Nursing education: foundations of practice excellence. Philadelphia: FA Davis; 2007. p. 213–6.
6. Prideaux D. The emperor's new clothes: from objectives to outcomes. Med Educ 2000;34:168–9.

7. Shreiber R, Bannister E. Challenges of teaching in an emancipatory curriculum. J Nurs Educ 2002;41(1):41–5.
8. Krathwohl DR, Bloom BS, Masia BB. Taxonomy of educational objectives, book 2: affective domain. New York: Longman; 1964.
9. Dave RH. Developing and writing behavioral objectives. Tucson (AZ): Educational Innovators Press; 1975.
10. Simpson EJ. The classification of educational objectives in the psychomotor domain. Washington, DC: Gryphon House; 1972.
11. Harrow A. A taxonomy of psychomotor domain: a guide for developing behavioral objectives. New York: David McKay; 1972.
12. Packard MJ. The new Bloom's taxonomy: an overview for family and consumer services. Journal of Family and Consumer Sciences Education 2007;25(1):45–55.
13. Spanner E. Historical introduction to the scientific publications program of the Academy of Natural Sciences. The Academy of Natural Sciences 150. Available at: http://www.acnatsci.org/library/scipubs/history/html. Accessed April 7, 2011.
14. Anderson L, Krathwohl DE. A taxonomy for learning teaching and assessing: a revision of Bloom's taxonomy of educational objectives [Abridged]. New York: Addison Wesley Longman, Inc.; 2001.
15. Larkin BG, Burton KJ. Evaluating a case study using Bloom's taxonomy of education. AORN J 2008;88(30):390–402.
16. Marzano RJ, Kendall JS. The new taxonomy of educational objectives. 2nd edition. Thousand Oaks (CA): Corwin Press; 2007.
17. Bloom BS, Engelhart MD, Furst EJ, et al, editors. Taxonomy of educational objectives: the classification of educational goals. Handbook I: cognitive domain. New York: David McKay; 1956.
18. Amer A. Reflections on Bloom's revised taxonomy. Electron J Res Educ Psychol 2006;8(4):213–30.
19. Krathwohl D. A revision of Bloom's taxonomy: an overview. Theory Into Practice 2002;41(4):212–8.
20. Furst E. Bloom's taxonomy: philosophical and educational issues. In: Anderson L, Sosniak L, editors. Bloom's taxonomy: a forty-year retrospective. Chicago: The National Society for the Study of Education; 1994. p. 28–40.
21. Kreitzer A, Madaus G. Empirical investigations of the hierarchal structure of the taxonomy. In: Anderson L, Sosniak L, editors. Bloom's taxonomy: a forty-year retrospective. Chicago: The National Society for the Study of Education; 1994. p. 64–81.
22. Anderson L. Revised Bloom's taxonomy. Paper presented at North Carolina Cancer and Technical Education Curriculum Development Training. Raleigh (NC), May, 2006.
23. Bransford J, Brown A, Cocking R. How people learn: brain, mind, experience, and school. Washington, DC: National Academy Press; 1999.
24. Gronlund NE. How to write and use instructional objectives. 6th edition. Upper Saddle River (NJ): Prentice Hall; 2000.
25. Huba ME, Freed JE. Learning-centered assessment on college campuses: shifting the focus from teaching to learning. Boston: Allyn and Bacon; 2000. p. 62.
26. Mertler CA. Teaching and assessment: the instructional process. In: Classroom assessment: a practical guide for educators. Los Angeles (CA): Pyrczak Publishing; 2003. p. 21–48.

Assessing Learning Styles: Practical Tips for Patient Education

Theresa Inott, MSN, RN*, Betsy B. Kennedy, MSN, RN

KEYWORDS

- Patient education • Patient teaching • Learning styles
- Teaching strategies • Adult learning

Nurses occupy a critical role in patient education. To facilitate and support patient and family decision-making, and to improve health outcomes, nurses are expected to possess expert instructional skills. The increasing complexity of patient needs and nursing responsibilities necessitates practical solutions for making the most of patient teaching encounters. Assessing patient learning style in combination with the context in which learning occurs allows for an individualized approach that incorporates teaching modalities to maximize patient learning. Understanding how and why adults learn and the necessary dimensions of assessment provides a foundation for application of a framework to organize patient teaching and facilitate learning.

MOTIVATION FOR LEARNING

The adult learner is one that has developed a pattern of behaviors, thoughts, and feelings that influence how teaching is received and learning is experienced. Knowles[1] theorized that adult learners are characterized by autonomy, rigidity, goal and relevancy orientation, practicality, and experience. Adults enter into learning for the purpose of change in skills, behavior, knowledge, or attitudes; therefore, this motivation is a key factor in initiating education. Awareness by the patient of the importance of what is being learned is essential because adults are motivated by their personal *need* to know the information. The individual must view the personal application of what is being taught within the context that it is occurring.

Logically, in health care settings, the adult patient is predominantly motivated to learn about what most concerns them. Thus, the internal needs of the individual present moments of readiness.[2] Collaborating with the patient to assess for primary and secondary concerns fosters the environment of teaching and learning through mutual

The authors have nothing to disclose.

Vanderbilt University School of Nursing, 311 Godchaux Hall, 21st Avenue South, Nashville, TN 37240, USA

* Corresponding author.

E-mail address: theresa.inott@vanderbilt.edu

goal setting and clarity of expectations. Involvement of the patient in this assessment and planning improves the likelihood of active participation in the learning process because it meets the need of the adult learner to be self-directed. Understanding the adult patient as a learner who is motivated by autonomy also requires consideration of their previous learning and life experiences when assessing their learning style.

Assessment of previous learning experience is valuable in determining the impact of past positive or negative events. Positive encounters will offer a constructive path toward similar approaches. Negative occurrences if not identified can be detrimental to new learning. Adults bring a rich life history to teaching and learning opportunities. In approaching new situations reflections on past experiences assist in current problem-solving.[3] To acquire new knowledge, adult learners need to apply new information to previous familiar events and have the foresight to determine its personal usefulness in the future.

DIMENSIONS OF ASSESSMENT

Just as assessment is the crucial first step in implementing the nursing process it is also the important initial stage in determining readiness to learn. This vital phase is often the most neglected or ignored aspect when preparing for patient teaching. Personal attributes that may influence learning style should be determined and incorporated into the plan.[4] Holistic assessment, which includes many factors, is necessary for developing effective teaching strategies that meet the unique needs of the individual's learning style. Physical, emotional, social, cultural, environmental, and learning characteristics must all be considered when determining readiness for patient teaching.

Physiologic conditions may affect the patient's cognitive abilities of attention, information processing, and memory. Acquisition and use of information initially requires the ability to maintain attention, followed by intellectual mental activities required for recall of information. Sensory impairments, physical limitations, and effects of medications may diminish the patient's capability to fully use their usual learning style.

Within the health care setting, situational psychological states such as anxiety, depression, fear, and acceptance or denial of illness are some of the factors that influence capacity and motivation to learn. The ability of the patient to concentrate is significantly affected while they are hospitalized.[5] At a time when the need for learning is great, these common mental stressors can significantly impair comprehension and alter the patient's usual style of learning.

In the United States, literacy is equated with the ability to read and write English. In their most recent 2003 report, the US Department of Education detailed that 28% of Americans possess very basic literacy skills with an additional 14% falling below the basic level.[6] The average adult American reads at the eighth to ninth grade level, and one of five read at the fifth grade level or below. Literacy is not necessarily a reflection of educational level. Chang and Kelly[7] support this opinion, maintaining that reading skills for many people are appreciably below completed level of formal schooling. Conversely, Wingard[4] makes note of the fact that a substantial proportion of patients have above-average literacy proficiency. Evaluation of literacy is imperative for planning strategies that address basic individualized teaching-learning needs.

Values and beliefs that are unique to each patient are determined by the individual's cultural norms. Culture is much broader than race or country of origin.[8] Generally, culture is identified by shared practices and traditions of a similar group. Using this characterization, differences in experience, sexual orientation, gender, and age would be considered as cultural distinctions. Learning styles are understandably influenced by these principles. In addition to attending to the innate needs of the adult learner, the nurse must be culturally sensitive to particular perceptions of illness, health beliefs, family roles, and communication when assessing learning styles of diverse patients. This requires nurses to ascertain as much information as possible about the explicit ways of the lives of the patient's in their care. It is vital to consider individuals and not assume they adhere to all traditions inherent to their cultures customs.[7] Personal nuances must be carefully evaluated as accurate appraisal is valuable in determining the unique needs of the patient as well as the patient's readiness to learn.

The physical setting within the health care facility, often seemingly benign to the nurse who is accustomed to the setting, can affect learning as well. Temperature, lighting, noise level, and lack of privacy are a few examples of environmental factors that may be distracting and uncomfortable obstacles. System barriers may also be problematic, such as lack of sufficient time, inadequate preparation or experiences of the nurse, and limited availability of resources. **Box 1** summarizes factors influencing patient learning styles that should be assessed and addressed in planning and implementation of teaching.

LEARNING STYLES

Although there are numerous theories of learning, Fleming and Mills'[9] VARK theory of learning styles is very conducive to patient education. The acronym VARK represents the Visual, Aural, Read or Write, and Kinesthetic sensory modalities used for learning. The theory also takes into consideration that the majority of individuals may be multimodal. The four styles of learning are expanded below.

Visual (V)

The visual preference includes the depiction of information in diagrams, charts, graphs, and symbols that can be used to represent what could have been presented in words. Visual learners prefer information processing through illustrations, pictures, and words. If nurses give verbal instruction to visual learners, it should also be provided in printed form.

Aural or Auditory (A)

The aural mode describes a preference for information processing through hearing. Patients with a preference for this modality learn best through discussion, groups, speaking, web chat, and talking things through. They prefer the spoken word and may read written materials aloud to themselves. Nurses should plan to verbally explain care instructions and minimize distractions that might interfere with hearing.

Read or Write (R)

This category of learners is sometimes difficult to distinguish from visual learners, but refers to a preference for information displayed specifically as words. Patients in this category prefer text, reading, and writing.

Kinesthetic (K)

The kinesthetic or tactile mode refers to a perceptual preference for experience and practice, which may be simulated or real. The sense of touch facilitates learning through actual doing or manipulation. Engaging the patient in a physical activity enhances the learning experience.

Many patients may be multimodal, or equally strong in information processing not limited to one mode. It is tempting to simply design teaching strategies that incorporate all learning styles, but this can be confusing and less effective than individualizing

Box 1
Dimensions of assessment

Biophysical

    Age

    Visual acuity

    Hearing

    Pain

    Fatigue

    Manual dexterity

    Medications

Psychological

    Anxiety

    Defensiveness

    Coping style

    Stress levels

    Adaptation to illness

    Life outlook

Social

    Perception of setting

    Perception of learning experiences

    Education

    Literacy

    Occupation

    Income

    Housing

    Dietary patterns

    Sleep patterns

    Exercise

    Sexuality

Cultural

    Language and communication

    Religious beliefs

    Cultural traditions

    Timing

Environmental

    Learning styles

    Learning environment

Data from Phillips LD. Patient education: understanding the process to maximize time and outcomes. J Intr Nurs 1999;22:19–35.

strategies to meet patient needs within their context. A variety of methods, modes, and materials should be available, but the best opportunities for learning are created from an awareness and use of individual learning styles. A summary of the VARK learning style characteristics and suggested teaching strategies are presented in **Table 1**.

Assessment for the VARK guide to learning styles involves answering simple questions about preferences for learning. The easily accessible Web site, located at http://www.vark-learn.com, asks only 16 questions, which are then analyzed to determine the test takers favored learning style. The instrument is available in several languages.

It is important to remember that preferences are not necessarily strengths and the mode a patient reports as favored may not really be the mode in which the patient learns best. The nurse must be flexible in methods and vigilant in evaluation for determining congruence between preferences and learning outcomes. Additionally, most nurses will approach patient teaching methods in the ways with which they themselves are most comfortable, even if it is not the most effective method or the patient's preference. Using a model to guide the educational process from assessment to evaluation is similar to what nurses do when providing patient care. This contributes to positive learning outcomes.

THE ASSURE MODEL

The ASSURE model, originally developed by Heinich and colleagues[10] for instructional design purposes, is useful in organizing the progression of patient teaching and is similar to the familiar nursing process. The ASSURE (Assess, Diagnose, Plan, Implement, Evaluate) model includes analysis of the learner; statement of objectives; selection of media, materials, and methods; implementation of methods; learner performance; and evaluation of the teaching and learning process. Applying this systematic approach to patient teaching is useful for maximizing efforts and benefits in education, and ensures emphasis on analysis. An overview of this model is presented in **Table 2**.

Table 1
VARK learning styles, characteristics, and teaching strategies

Learning Style	Characteristics	Teaching Strategies
Visual	• Preference for written instructions, photographs and illustrations to view	• Variety of interesting options • Attractive, easy-to-read handouts • Use of technological variety
Aural (Auditory)	• Preference for listening to instruction and discussion • Remembers through verbal repetition	• Variations in presentations of tone, pitch, and speed • Multimedia that uses speech and sounds such as audio recordings
Reading	• Preference for written instructions and materials	• Provide handouts • Required and suggested readings
Kinesthetic/Tactile	• Preference for getting physically involved • Remembers by doing or experiencing	• Encourage movement • Use of multimedia • Tactile activities • Return demonstrations

From Russell S. An overview of adult-learning processes. Uro Nurs 2006;26:349–52, 370; with permission.

Table 2 The ASSURE model		
A	Analyze	• Determine what the patient needs to learn • Determine the characteristics of the learner • Determine the learning style of the patient
S	State Objectives	• Outline the goals for learning • Focus on the patient as learner and as partner in creating goals for learning • Consider the circumstances for learning • Determine the level of mastery required
S	Select, Modify, Design Media and Materials	• Decide which tools will be most appropriate for learning • Determine the best ways to facilitate learning based on the stated goals and analysis
U	Utilize Materials	• Preview the materials, prepare the materials, environment, patient, and provide the experience • Employ the various tools in patient teaching
R	Require Learner Performance	• Decide how the patient will demonstrate evidence of learning • Have the patient demonstrate evidence of knowledge gained
E	Evaluate and Re-evaluate	• Evaluate the patient's demonstration of learning • Evaluate the methods, media, and materials used • Evaluate teacher (nurse) performance

From Heinich, Molenda, Russell, et al. Instructional media and technologies for learning. 7th edition. New Jersey: Merrill Prentice Hall; 2002; with permission.

Understanding the patient and the context for learning through assessment and analysis is the essential first step in the process of facilitating learning. Neglecting this step in the interest of saving time and using a generic patient teaching scenario can adversely affect learning and ultimately impair the educational outcome.

Choosing the appropriate resources is dependent upon analysis of not only learning styles, but also setting, abilities, prior knowledge, and desired competencies. Stating the specific objectives and desired outcomes, developed in tandem with the patient, focuses the teaching on meeting the needs and motives of each encounter.

When selecting media, methods, and materials to facilitate patient learning, the nurse bases decisions on information learned in learning style assessment. Depending on the specific topic, materials for patient teaching may be limited or abundant. Demonstration, pamphlets, other print resources, videos, Internet resources, audio recordings, illustrations, games, or other electronic media are commonly used for patient education. Additionally, opportunities may exist for group or individualized teaching. The nurse determines the best approaches and media combinations available for use with the specific patient, setting, and goals.

After selection of appropriate materials, methods, or media for use in objective, focused patient teaching, the next step is application. Implementing the plan for teaching in collaboration with the patient also involves familiarity with the chosen methods. The nurse must be comfortable and confident in the content and chosen approach for patient teaching. Getting the patient involved in the process reduces passivity and makes the patient an active participant.

Expertise in patient teaching requires reflection by the nurse. Evaluating the level of patient participation, how well they learned in relation to the stated goals and objectives, and the usefulness of the methods and materials used is an important step useful in determining the need for reassessment of learning styles because it illuminates barriers that may have influenced the process. Reflection on the effectiveness of patient teaching requires consideration of evidence that learning has taken place and that it is has improved patient knowledge, health outcomes such as symptom management, and self-care skills.[11] More recently, patient teaching outcome studies have also included cost-effectiveness of patient education methods, patient satisfaction with teaching and subsequent quality of life, and hospital readmissions.[11]

ADDRESSING BARRIERS

Failure to assess the learning style characteristics of individual patients is a common barrier in planning and implementation of patient teaching. The VARK model offers a simple, easy-to-use guide for evaluation of patient preferences. Although the inclusion of more than one approach might be confusing for some, most people possess multimodal preferences. Skills of both the patient and nurse are often enhanced by the inclusion of more than one approach. A variety of methods and media that highlight more than one learning preference should be used whenever possible to meet the most universal needs of individuals.[2–4] Though we may have the ability to use multiple tools and formats that address favored learning styles, it is vital to first assess the individual patient's needs, readiness, and capabilities.

As a significant number of Americans fall within the category of basic or below-basic literacy skills, the majority of teaching tools should be designed with this fact in mind. Printed materials are routinely used with other teaching strategies. To be understood by the majority of patients, written documents and other modes of patient education should be developed at the fifth grade reading level.[7]

Basic communication may inadvertently block the potential for learning. The vocabulary and jargon often used by health care providers can be an obstacle. Additionally, lack of respect may be communicated and perceived if the nurse does not pronounce the patient or family's name correctly or chooses to addresses them by first name rather than surname. Illness and hospitalization are particularly stressful occasions. For those to whom English is a second language, understanding may be particularly difficult and usual learning styles may be altered to accommodate language issues.

The most noticeable barriers to assessing learning style and abilities are those associated with the needs of a culturally diverse population. The nurse must reflect on his or her own health beliefs and practices and determine if personal views have influenced the assessment of learning style and choice of teaching strategies. Coming from a background that is very different from the patient's background may result in poor communication and some behaviors may be perceived by the patient as offensive. For example, the family roles within a given culture may require that teaching is undertaken with a specific relative or group. To ensure that health behaviors will be implemented, the learning style of the key members must be addressed. Understanding the health care practices of the individual and family is essential. Within some cultures, the need for further education is not apparent if symptoms have lessened.[7] This practice could hinder motivation to learn, because adult learners must perceive the need to solve a problem and understand how the information will be helpful to them.

Patient motivation is determined by existing physical and emotional restrictions, the immediate need to know information, and overall level of confidence. To address the barriers related to physical and emotional impairment, the nurse is understandably limited. Acknowledging the likelihood of these influences allows for adjustments in assessment, planning, and implementation. For instance, if a known disability exists, such as visual or hearing impairment, pain, or anxiety, alterations inherent to such circumstances must be considered. Adult learners are self-directed and self-regulated. This requires that the information being taught has personal meaning to the individual adult leaner. For some, this may require that the nurse is able to identify the teachable moment and convince the patient of the importance of learning particular details regarding their illness and/or recovery. Confidence is generated by several factors: the ability to meet learning goals, the challenge of learning large amounts of information, and the comfort of operating from their personal learning preference or style. Adult learners need to be a part of the planning process in order to be motivated. This includes the development of achievable and relevant mutually valued goals.[7] To meet this requirement, abundant information can be broken down into small easily achievable amounts of learning designed to first meet short-term goals. This will build confidence because the adult learner is able to master the new knowledge.

CONCLUSION

The goal of patient teaching is to address patient knowledge, behaviors, attitudes, and skills so that they are able to assume responsibility for their own care.[12]

Assessment is the essential first step in developing teaching strategies for individual patients and the process of education. Appraisal of learning style helps to determine a teaching approach that meets the true needs of adult patients. Use of the VARK learning style assessment tool with added assessment of the multiple dimensions influencing the individual learner provides vital information for planning the context for knowledge acquisition in the learning-teaching relationship.

REFERENCES

1. Knowles MS. Modern practice of adult education: from pedagogy to andragogy. 2nd edition. New York: Cambridge Books; 1980. p. 37.
2. Russell SS. An overview of adult-learning processes. Urol Nurs 2006;26:349–52.
3. Weaver D. Understanding the learning process. Nursing Residential Care 2010; 12:470–2.
4. Wingard R. Patient education and the nursing process: meeting the patient's needs. Nephrol Nurs J 2005;32:211–4.
5. Rafii F, Shahpoorian F, Azarbadd M. The reality of learning self-care needs during hospitalization: patients' and nurses' perceptions. Self-Care, Dependent-Care & Nursing 2008;16:34–9.
6. The National Assessment of Adult Literacy (NAAL, 2011). A first look at the literacy of America's adults in the 21st century. Available at: http://nces.ed.gov/naal. Accessed March 23, 2011.
7. Chang M, Kelly A. Patient education: addressing cultural diversity and health literacy issues. Urol Nurs 2007;27:411–7.
8. Stokes L, Flowers N. Multicultural education in nursing. In: Billings DM, Halstead JA, editors. Teaching in nursing: a guide for faculty. St Louis (MO): Saunders Elsevier; 2009. p. 268–82.
9. Fleming ND, Mills C. VARK a guide to learning styles 2002. 2010. Available at: http://www.vark-learn.com/English/index.asp. Accessed November 9, 2010.
10. Heinich R, Molenda M, Russell J, et al. Instructional media and technologies for learning. 7th edition. New Jersey: Merrill Prentice Hall; 2002.
11. Oermann MH. How effective is your patient teaching? J Wound Ostomy Continence Nurs 2003;30:122–5.
12. Phillips LD. Patient education: understanding the process to maximize time and outcomes. J Intraven Nurs 1999;22:19–35.

Promoting Health Literacy: A Nursing Imperative

Carolyn I. Speros, DNSc, APRN

KEYWORDS

• Health literacy • Patient education • Health promotion
• Health communication • Literacy • Nursing

Imagine that you are in a foreign country in which the spoken and written language is completely unfamiliar to you. You suddenly develop severe abdominal pain and realize that you must be evaluated by a medical professional. You cannot interpret the signs that direct you to the emergency room of the hospital. Everyone around you speaks his or her own language and no one takes the time to ask if you understand. You are asked multiple questions that you are unable to translate or comprehend. You are handed several pieces of paper that are incomprehensible and require your signature and consent. Your pain is intensifying throughout the duration of the process. Imagine the confusion, frustration, and panic that you feel. Unfortunately, in the United States, this scenario is all too real for the approximately 90 million Americans who struggle with reading because they are victims of the silent epidemic of low health literacy.

Nearly 9 out of 10 adults in the United States experience difficulty understanding and using basic health information provided to them in hospitals, clinics, and physicians' offices, or through media outlets such as television and the web.[1-3] Health literacy is a relatively new concept that came to the attention of public health researchers in the early 1990s. As the association between literacy, health outcomes, and health disparities became evident, a groundswell of research and academic work in the medical and public health arenas has been devoted to investigating strategies that promote health literacy in vulnerable populations. Nurses play a critical role in facilitating the communication processes that are associated with promoting health literacy. Assessing individual motivators, identifying barriers to comprehension, communicating clearly, making health information readable and accessible, adapting the message to the cultural and linguistic needs of the patient, promoting health decision-making, and evaluating comprehension are basic health literacy promotion strategies that nurses must use to facilitate patient understanding and empowerment. This article explores the concept of health literacy and its relationship to patient

---

The author has nothing to disclose.
University of Memphis, Loewenberg School of Nursing, Newport Hall, Memphis, TN 38152, USA
E-mail address: csperos@memphis.edu

Nurs Clin N Am 46 (2011) 321–333
doi:10.1016/j.cnur.2011.05.007
0029-6465/11/$ – see front matter © 2011 Elsevier Inc. All rights reserved.

education and communication. Practical strategies that the nurse can use to assess, communicate with, and evaluate comprehension in patients with low literacy skills will be provided.

WHAT IS HEALTH LITERACY?

The conceptual definitions of health literacy have evolved over time. Most agree that health literacy means that an individual has the capacity to read, understand, and act on health information. The landmark publications of *Healthy People 2010*[4] and the Institute of Medicine's (IOM) *Health Literacy: A Prescription to End Confusion* define health literacy in a similar way: "The degree to which individuals have the capacity to obtain, process, and understand basic health information and services needed to make appropriate health decisions."[1(p32)] Health literacy is viewed as a set of individual capacities that allow the patient to acquire, process, and use new health-related information. A health literate person is one who can successfully apply the skills of reading and writing, speaking and listening, computation, and comprehension within a health context. For example, a health literate person has the capacity and the necessary set of cognitive skills and physical abilities to read labels on prescription bottles, compute the correct dose of medicine to take each day, complete health insurance forms, know where and how often to go for health screenings, or give an informed consent. Many public health experts believe that adequate health literacy is a personal asset that positively influences an individual's health.[5] Inadequate or low health literacy is considered a health and safety risk which must be assessed for and managed in the clinical setting.[6] By improving people's access to health information and their capacity to interpret and use it effectively, health literacy is essential to informed decision-making.

The broadest definition of health literacy is promulgated by the World Health Organization (WHO): "Health literacy has been defined as the cognitive and social skills which determine the motivation and ability of individuals to gain access to, understand, and use information in ways that promote and maintain good health. Health literacy means more than being able to read pamphlets and make appointments. By improving people's access to health information, and their capacity to use it effectively, health literacy is critical to empowerment."[7] The WHO expands the perspective of health literacy to a larger economic, social, and political context. It speaks to the importance of a population's collective level of health literacy as a determinant of the health of the community-at-large.

Health literacy is dynamic and influenced by multiple individual, cultural, and social factors.[8] An individual's level of health literacy evolves over one's life, and is impacted by education, aging, social interactions, language, culture, and life experiences with health and illness.[8–11] Baker[12] suggests that health literacy is also directly influenced by the communication skills of the clinician and the complexities of the system in which that care is provided. Consequently, nurses must be cognizant of the direct impact that they have on a patient's level of health literacy during every patient encounter. Each patient presents with a certain capacity for understanding and using health information. To effectively promote health literacy, accommodations must be made on the nurse's part to make information accessible and clearly understood.

WHO IS AT RISK?

Inadequate health literacy affects people of all ages, races, socioeconomic situations, and educational levels. However, the impact of low health literacy as it relates to poor health outcomes and higher costs disproportionately affects lower socioeconomic and minority groups.[13] Identifying patients at risk for misunderstandings and potential errors in care before and after discharge is essential to the safe and ethical practice of nursing.

Patients with low health literacy are often difficult to identify. Because health literacy requires multiple complex cognitive and social skills in addition to reading, patients at risk may be excellent readers, highly educated, or affluent members of society. A significant number of people struggle in today's complex health care environment to understand medical terminology and concepts that are outside of the context of their usual work or social settings. It is for this reason that assessments of health literacy cannot be based on generalizations, stereotyping, or simply looking at the way a patient presents in the hospital or clinic setting.[14] All patients should be purposefully assessed for inadequate health literacy. This can be accomplished by incorporating a key question in the patient's history, recognizing behavioral cues that are often associated with low health literacy, or identifying those who fall within a high-risk category identified through literacy and social science research.

Many clinicians have found that the most expeditious way of assessing a patient's risk for inadequate health literacy is to add a specific question about the patient's reliance on and comfort with reading to the health history interview. After asking typical questions in the social history about the patient's occupation and education, the nurse might ask, "Do you enjoy reading?," "What do you enjoy reading?," "Where do you typically go to get health information?," or "What is the best way for you to learn new things about your illness or your health?" An open-ended question similar to these establishes a tone of support for the poor reader, and can lead into a discussion about alternative methods of providing information beyond those that require the patient to read.

Recent research in the area of screening patients for low literacy has identified two key questions that are sensitive for detecting limited literacy skills in patients. Morris and colleagues[15] developed the Single Item Literacy Screener (SILS) that poses the one question as a screen, "How often do you need to have someone help when you read instructions, pamphlets, or other written material from your doctor or pharmacy?" (positive answers are "sometimes," "often," or "always"). Another informal screening question, "How confident do you feel in filling out medical forms by yourself?" (positive answers are "somewhat," "a little bit," or "not at all") was also found to be reasonably successful in identifying patients at risk for low literacy.[16] Either of these questions can easily be incorporated in the initial assessment interview to identify those patients who might be at risk for low health literacy.

The Newest Vital Sign (NVS) developed by Weiss and colleagues[17] is a short assessment screening test that can be quickly administered to patients in a clinical setting. The test is available in English and Spanish and takes about 3 minutes to administer. The NVS is designed to screen for the patient's general literacy level, numeracy skills, and comprehension of health-related written material. Patients are asked to read a nutrition label. The clinician then asks the patient six questions about how they would act on the information. Patients who answer less than four of the questions correctly are considered at risk for low health literacy. The NVS is available online at no cost from the US Department of Health and Human Services' Health Resources and Services Administration Web site at http://pilot.train.hrsa.gov/uhc/pdf/module_02_job_aid_vital_sign.pdf.

Nurses must realize that patients may not always admit to having problems with reading because of the stigma associated with limited literacy. Poor readers often overestimate their ability to read, are ashamed to admit that they cannot read, or adopt certain behaviors that compensate for their inability to read.[18] One study found that up to 75% of patients who read at or below the fifth grade level report that they read "well" or "very well."[19] The astute nurse should assess for behaviors commonly used by poor readers to mask their inability to read. For example, patients may take a written handout, place it on the bedside table without reading it and say that they will read it at a later time. They may say that they want to show it to their spouse or child at the evening visit without looking at it. They may ask the nurse to read the information to them because they left their glasses at home. They may hesitate when filling out their registration form and leave several questions blank, or ask the nurse to complete a health history checklist for them. Poor readers read slowly, skip over unfamiliar words, read only the first sentence in a paragraph, interpret words literally, look only at the visuals, and tire easily when reading. Some suggest that the patient be asked to read a paragraph or important sentence from a health information piece aloud as the nurse watches for these clues to poor reading. Care must be taken to avoid setting a patient up for failure or embarrassment if this method of assessing for literacy is used. When observing any "red flags" or behavioral cues associated with poor reading skills, the nurse should use alternative teaching methods that are specifically designed for low literate learners.

There are several more formal instruments available that measure the patient's ability to recognize medical words and comprehend health-related text. These include the Rapid Estimate of Adult Literacy in Medicine (REALM),[20] the Short Assessment of Health Literacy for Spanish-Speaking Adults (SAHLSA),[21] the Short Test of Functional Health Literacy in Adults (s-TOFHLA),[22] and the Wide-Range Achievement Test, Level IV.[23] Most experts in the field of health literacy believe that these longer, more formal assessments of health literacy should be reserved for research. They are more time consuming to administer in a typical patient encounter, and yield little more insight into the needs of low literacy patients than the simple screens that have been mentioned above.

The US Department of Education conducted the National Assessment of Adult Literacy (NAAL)[24] in 2003 to measure the scope and breadth of literacy in American adults. At the urging of social scientists and health service researchers with *Healthy People 2010*,[4] health-related reading and comprehension items were included in the survey. The NAAL was the first large-scale national literacy assessment designed to measure the prevalence of health literacy in American adults. Data from the NAAL identified seven groups who were at higher risk for low health literacy.[2] These groups included the elderly, those who did not complete high school, members of ethnic minorities, and people who spoke a language other than English in their home. Unemployed persons, those with limited income, and individuals on Medicaid were also more likely to have limited health literacy. Although individuals within each of each of these groups may certainly function at a high level of health literacy, the nurse should use universal precautions for health literacy during all interactions with patients who fall within these seven groups.

STRATEGIES TO PROMOTE HEALTH LITERACY

Communication that is purposeful and patient-centered is essential to reaching patients with low health literacy. The responsible nurse who works with patients in today's complex health care environment must learn and believe that telling is not teaching, and that patient understanding cannot simply be assumed. Safe, quality nursing care can only be provided within a supportive and shame-free learning environment in which clear communication is intentionally used. Patient teaching materials and strategies must be specifically designed for low literacy patients, and nurses must

constantly validate that the intended message is accurately heard, processed, and understood by each patient. **Box 1** summarizes the evidence-based communication strategies that have been shown to promote health literacy in patients.

Create a Shame-free Environment

Being hospitalized is an emotionally charged experience for patients and their families. Fear, confusion, distrust, loneliness, and anxiety are common feelings that patients experience during an illness and hospitalization. Patients with low health literacy often feel shame and intimidation in the patient role because of the stigma associated with being unable to read and understand medical words and practices.[28,29] It is easy for nurses and other health care providers to forget that the daily routines and "language" of the hospital, which are second nature to them, are strange, foreign, and disorienting to patients. To create a supportive and shame-free environment that promotes health literacy, nurses must foster a respectful and caring atmosphere in which honesty, open dialog, and questions are encouraged.

Navigating the expectations, policies, procedures, and practices within a complex medical environment has been cited by many patients as the most frustrating and frightening aspect of being hospitalized.[14,30] Nurses must remain sensitive to the importance of frequently orienting the patient to their surroundings, daily activities on the unit, and nursing care routines. Simple explanations of "how things work around here" help ease a patient's anxiety and create an environment in which patients are more receptive to communication and teaching. The nurse might consider constructing in clear language a "frequently asked questions" handout about unit processes. Pens or pencils should be provided to encourage patients to add their own questions. The staff can then review the questions and answers with the patient orally, creating an opportunity to promote open dialog. Before leaving, the nurse should use the "teach back" approach to evaluate understanding. Can the patient tell the nurse what will be happening next, when, and how long it will take? Can the patient tell the nurse what tests are planned, what they are for, and what will occur?

Empathy (understanding and validating a patient's feelings) is a critical element of supportive communication. Being empathetic demonstrates caring and concern, and thus promotes patient trust. A trusting relationship between the patient and the nurse creates an environment in which patients can get help and information without feeling stigmatized or intimidated when asking questions. Empathy can be manifested by saying, "It can be overwhelming when so much information is given to you while you are sick," or "Medical words are not very easy to understand. Lots of patients find this confusing."

Patients with limited health literacy prefer clear communication with short words and sentences that cover only essential, need-to-know information. Multiple studies have demonstrated the wide gap between the reading grade level of signage, postings, brochures, and pamphlets used in the hospital setting and the reading and comprehension levels of most patients.[31,32] Patients struggle with completing written forms and answering the myriad of questions asked during admission to the hospital and nursing unit. They often have multiple questions before discharge about follow-up and what to do at home. Knowing this, the nurse who is sensitive to the needs of patients with low health literacy will consistently do the following:

- Verbally introduce yourself and explain your role. Do not expect patients to be able to read the name on your nametag or lab coat. Reintroduce yourself each day that you come into the patient's room.

Box 1
Strategies to promote health literacy

Create a shame-free environment

- Encourage questions
- Show respect, helpfulness, caring attitude
- Orient to surroundings, nursing care routines, people on unit
- Provide "frequently-asked questions" handout and review orally
- Convey empathy and reassurance
- Assist in completing forms
- Speak slowly and distinctly
- Ensure patient privacy when talking
- Ask patient to share what was heard after physician's visit and clarify
- Teach patients to ask:
  - What is my main problem?
  - What do I need to do about the problem?
  - Why is it important for me to do this?
- Invite a family member or friend
- Offer note pad and pencil
- Simplify self-care and treatment regimens as much as possible
- Be positive and supportive

Use clear purposeful communication

- Intentionally speak clearly, distinctly
- Use plain, everyday language
- Avoid medical and technical jargon
- Limit key points to three or fewer
- Face patient when speaking
- Put information in a familiar context
- Repeat and review key points
- Avoid medical concept and categorical words
- Be specific and concrete; avoid words that require inferences
- Use vocabulary that is familiar to the patient
- Define new health care and medical terms
- Consistently use same terms
- Conclude with a summary of key points

Communicate in a patient-centered manner

- Identify patient's personal motivators
- Assess unique interests and activities
- Address patient's main concern
- Link new information to past experiences
- Assess what is already known

- Be sensitive to age and cultural mores
- Use active voice and personalize the message
- Accommodate visual, hearing and cognitive changes in the elderly

Reinforce the spoken word

- Use a variety of methods: photographs, audio, and drawings
- Select or create only highly readable written materials
  - Summarize key points in the first paragraph
  - Put a heading before each section
  - Use 14 point, plain font with uppercase and lowercase letters
  - Use short sentences of fewer than eight words
  - Write at the fifth grade level
  - Number steps in sequence
  - Use black ink on white or buff paper with plenty of white space
  - Bold key points
  - Use simple line drawings or pictographs
  - Summarize key points at the end
- Read aloud written forms and handouts

Verify understanding

- Ask "What questions do you have?"
- Use teach-back technique
- Ask patient to paraphrase instructions
- Observe return demonstration and provide feedback
- "Tell me how you will do this once you get home?"
- Observe patient teaching others in your presence and give feedback

Data from Refs.[14,25–27]

- Use open body language and make eye contact with the patient. Position yourself near the patient's bedside and face the patient while speaking. This position facilitates lip reading for patients who are hard of hearing.
- Be respectful, addressing the patient by their title and last name. Demonstrate a helpful and caring attitude.
- Reassure the patient that you welcome questions. Tell the patient that you do not mind repeating anything that has been said.
- Offer all patients help in completing forms. Sit beside the patient and read the form aloud. Be sure to minimize the chances of being overheard by others. The patient will be more likely to be open if the setting is private.
- Speak slowly and distinctly. Deepen the pitch of your voice. Elderly patients who are hard of hearing have trouble hearing high-pitched sounds. Speak in a normal volume.
- After a physician's visit, ask the patient to share with you in his or her own words what was heard. Clarify information that was not understood. Act as the patient's advocate to get access to more complete information if needed.

- Before discharge, read the discharge instructions to the patient. Pause frequently to encourage questions. Ask the patient to describe or demonstrate any procedures that need to be done in the patient's home after discharge.
- Write down the name of the provider, and the date, time and location of the first follow-up appointment and review the information with the patient. Offer to call and make the appointment for the patient.

Clear Purposeful Communication

Using clear communication purposefully is one of the most important ways that clinicians can reduce the health disparities related to inadequate health literacy.[25] Common errors that nurses and physicians make in communicating with patients include using jargon and technical words, overwhelming the patient with too much information, relying only on the spoken word, and failing to tailor the instructions to the unique motivators and goals of the patient.[33,34]

Patients with low health literacy often rely solely on the spoken word.[35] Therefore, verbal communication must be made intentionally clear. Nurses should speak slowly, use plain language with words that their own family members could understand, and avoid using medical and technical jargon. For example, the nurse should say "not cancer" rather than using the term "benign." Matching the clinician's vocabulary with the vocabulary of the patient has been shown to be effective in reaching a patient with low literacy skills because it allows the patient to cognitively relate to a common vocabulary and experience.[34,36]

To promote retention and recall, the amount of information given should be limited to three or fewer need-to-know key points. The content of the message should be directed at the action, skills, or behaviors that result in the desired health outcomes. The key points should be organized so that there is logical progression from simple to complex. Each cluster or "chunk" of information should require no more than 5 to 10 minutes to explain. Adequate time should be allowed for the patient to process the information. Early successes in mastering basic key points are empowering to the patient and create a foundation for more complex learning later. Repetition and review enhances knowledge acquisition and retention over time.

Patients with low health literacy have trouble processing abstract and nonspecific concepts and categorical words. Nurses should avoid using medical concept words, such as "factor," "referral," "avoid," or "active role." Categorical words commonly used in medical jargon, such as "generic," "hazardous," or "adverse," should be also be avoided. Words that require the patient to make inferences or judgments, such as "adequately," "routinely," "frequently," "often," or "as needed," are easily misunderstood and can lead to patient noncompliance.[34,36,37] Directions (particularly as they relate to medications and critical self care skills after discharge) should be provided using concrete and specific terms. For example, the nurse should tell the patient to "Take your yellow pill in the morning after breakfast and at night after a snack before going to bed," rather than "Take your high blood pressure pill twice a day."

Patient-Centered Communication

Literacy experts emphasize the importance of tailoring communication and teaching to what is valued, relevant, and meaningful to the patient.[14,18,27] Nurses should assess the activities and interests that are perceived by the patient as important to maintaining their functional independence and quality of life realistically within the parameters of the patient's health status ("What do you think most about doing after you go home?" or "What did you enjoy doing before you became sick?"). Once these internal motivators are identified, teaching can be individualized to focus on what the patient needs to know and do to reach their own unique goals. Many experts suggest that patients be asked what they already know about the topic ("What do you know about...?" or "Tell me what you have heard about...").[26] The patient's response to this question will often uncover the patient's main concern, misconceptions, or gaps in knowledge. Communication is most effective if it addresses the patient's main concern. The patient's perceived barriers to performing a prescribed activity or recommendation should be assessed. The nurse can then assist the patient in working through those barriers that *the patient* identifies as most challenging.

Reinforcing the Spoken Word

Clear purposeful verbal instructions may need to be reinforced with other teaching modalities, such as written handouts, brochures, written lists, and videos. When writing or selecting written materials to be used in the process of teaching patients with low literacy skills, do the following: (1) limit key points to one or two; (2) write legibly (printing preferred) allowing for adequate "white" space between words; (3) if using a printer, chose at least a 14-point, nonserif font such as Arial or Helvetica and consistently use that font style throughout; (4) use uppercase and lowercase text; (5) use bold letters (not italicized or all upper case) to emphasize key points; (6) use the active voice ("Rest with your lower legs elevated" rather than "You should elevate your legs when you rest"); (7) use words that are one or two syllables; (8) keep sentences short and succinct with fewer than eight words; (9) keep the reading level at fifth grade or below; and (10) use pictures generously.[14,18,36] Multiple studies have shown that the combination of pictographs and verbal instruction and pictures added to written text improved low literacy patients' recall and adherence to treatment recommendations.[38,39] Select visuals that clarify the key points of the content and portray the recommended actions visually. Pictures and illustrations should be age and culturally appropriate to the intended readers.

Verifying Understanding

Verifying and evaluating understanding is one of the most critical elements of effective communication with low literacy patients. Asking "What questions do you have?" is a good way to initiate a dialog. It suggests that questions are expected and empowers patients to get their questions answered. Care must be taken to avoid asking "Do you have any questions?" or "Do you understand?" Experience has shown that patients often answer "yes" to these questions even though they still have multiple questions and misconceptions about the content.

After the patient's questions have been answered, the "teach-back" technique should be used. This technique has been shown to be an effective method of verifying understanding in low literacy patients.[26] Teach-back involves asking patients to explain the intended message in their own words or demonstrate the target skill being taught, and then briefly explaining why you are asking. For example, the nurse might ask "I'd like for you to tell me how you might feel when you are coming down with low blood sugar so that I can be sure that what I have said to you is clear and makes sense," or "So that I can be sure that I have given you clear instructions, when your wife comes by tonight to visit and asks you what the nurse said, what will you tell her?" By using the teach-back method, the nurse communicates ownership and responsibility for teaching the patient effectively. If the patient cannot adequately explain the important aspects of the content or satisfactorily demonstrate the intended skill, then the nurse can focus on reviewing the content that was not learned. Studies have shown that using the teach-back method improves both patient comprehension and outcomes of care, and does not result in longer patient encounters.[14,33,40]

Table 1
Landmark initiatives at the national level in support of health literacy

Healthy People 2010 (2000)	Health objectives for the nation focused on HL
Priority Areas for National Action: Transforming Health Care Quality (IOM report) 2003	HL listed as a cross-cutting priority for health care organizations
Health Literacy: A Prescription to End Confusion (IOM report) 2004	Defined HL. Recommended governmental support and funding for research and HL initiatives. Recommended medical and nursing education programs incorporate HL in curricula and areas of competence.
Department of Education's National Assessment Adult Literacy (NAAL) (Results reported 2006)	Measured prevalence of inadequate HL in US
Surgeon General's Workshop on Improving Health Literacy (2006)	Initiated dialog about HL with public and private entities and the Surgeon General's office
Joint Commission Report, "What Did the Doctor Say?" (2007)	Established the link between HL, safety, and quality care
Plain Writing Act (2010)	Established that government documents issued to the public must be written clearly
Patient Protection and Affordable Care Act (2010)	Included HL as law in specified programs
National Action Plan to Improve Health Literacy (HHS) (2010)	Vision and goals set for a health literate society. Resources provided for communities to improve HL

Abbreviation: HL, health literacy.

HEALTH LITERACY UNIVERSAL PRECAUTIONS

Multiple agencies and experts in the area of health literacy recommend that universal precautions for low health literacy be implemented in all health care facilities.[13,41] "Universal precautions" means that specific actions should be taken which minimize the risk for everyone when it is unclear which patients may be affected with the problem.[42] Because of the widespread prevalence of inadequate health literacy and the difficulty in being able to determine which patients are at risk, it is recommended that nurses communicate with every patient as if he or she will have difficulty understanding what is said. The Joint Commission's[43] accreditation standards underscore the fundamental right of patients to receive information in ways that can be understood. Inadequate health literacy and ineffective communication place patients at greater risk of preventable adverse events. Promoting understanding enhances safety and health outcomes in all patients regardless of their level of health literacy.

SUMMARY

Over the past two decades, health policy experts, social scientists, and health researchers have given much needed attention to the evolving concept of health literacy.[44] Multiple reports, white papers, and federal initiatives are calling for a focus on clear communication and the use of evidence-based strategies that address the problem of low health literacy. **Table 1** lists the landmark publications and actions at the national level that support the promotion of health literacy as an integral part of safe quality health care in America.

It is imperative that nursing responds to the call of creating a health literate society by taking an active role in health literacy research, education, and promotion. Nurses are major players in a health care system that places significant reading and comprehension demands on patients and their families. It is essential that nurses understand the prevalence and presentation of low health literacy, acknowledge that it can be a significant barrier to safe and effective care, and commit to communicating more effectively and compassionately with those who struggle with the problem. Many adverse outcomes associated with low health literacy may be related to ineffective or poor nurse-patient communication. Evidence-based strategies that promote health literacy must be incorporated in every patient's plan of care and become part of the routine practice of nursing. Nurses have a professional and ethical obligation to communicate in a clear, purposeful way that addresses the unique information needs of each patient. Because knowledge is power and comprehension is empowering, the goal of all patient interactions should be to empower the patient to obtain, understand, and act on information that is needed for optimal health.

REFERENCES

1. Nielsen-Bohlman L, Panzer AM, Kindig DA, editors. Institute of medicine. Health literacy: a prescription to end confusion. Washington, DC: National Academies Press; 2004.
2. Kutner M, Greenberg E, Jin Y, et al. The health literacy of America's adults: results from the 2003 national assessment of adult literacy. Washington, DC: National Center for Educational Statistics; 2006; NCES–483.
3. Rudd RE. Health literacy skills of U.S. adults. Am J Health Behav 2007;31(Suppl 1): S8–18.
4. US Department of Health and Human Services. Healthy people 2010: national health promotion and disease prevention objectives. Washington, DC: US Department of Health and Human Services; 2000.
5. Nutbeam D. The evolving concept of health literacy. Soc Sci Med 2008;67(12): 2072–8.
6. Paasche-Orlow MK, Wolf MS. The causal pathways linking health literacy to health outcomes. Am J Health Behav 2007;31:S19–26.
7. World Health Organization. Track 2. Health literacy and health behaviour: 7th global conference on health promotion. Available at: http://www.who.int/healthpromotion/conferences/7gchp/track2/en/index.html. Accessed November 27, 2010.
8. Berkman ND, Davis TC, McCormack L. Health literacy: what is it? J Health Commun 2010;15(Suppl 2):9–19.
9. Zarcadoolas C, Pleasant AF, Greer DS. Advancing health literacy: a framework for understanding and action. San Francisco (CA): Jossey-Bass; 2006.
10. Speros CI. Health literacy: concept analysis. J Adv Nurs 2005;50(6):633–40.
11. Mancuso JM. Health literacy: a concept/dimensional analysis. Nurs Health Sci 2008;10:248–55.
12. Baker DW. The meaning and the measure of health literacy. J Gen Intern Med 2006;21(8):878–83.
13. US Department of Health and Human Services, Office of Disease Prevention and Health Promotion. National action plan to improve health literacy. Washington, DC: 2010. Available at: http://www.health.gov/communication/hlactionplan/. Accessed November 24, 2010.

14. Weiss BD. Health literacy: a manual for clinicians. 2nd editon. Chicago: American Medical Association Foundation; 2007.
15. Morris NS, MacLean CD, Chew LD, et al. The single item literacy screener: evaluation of a brief instrument to identify limited reading ability. BMC Fam Pract 2006;7:21.
16. Wallace LS, Rogers ES, Roskos SE, et al. Brief report: screening items to identify patients with limited health literacy skills. J Gen Intern Med 2006;21(8):874–7.
17. Weiss BD, Mays MZ, Martz W, et al. Quick assessment of literacy in primary care: the newest vital sign. Ann Fam Med 2005;3(6):514–22.
18. Cornett S. Assessing and addressing health literacy. Online J Issues Nurs 2009; 14(3):1–18.
19. Kirsch IS, Jungeblut A, Jenkins L, et al. Executive summary of adult literacy in America: A first look at the results of the national adult literacy survey. Washington, DC: National Center for Education Statistics, US Dept. of Education; 1993.
20. Davis TC, Long S, Jackson R, et al. Rapid estimate of adult literacy in medicine: a shortened screening instrument. Fam Med 1993;25:391–5.
21. Lee SY, Bender DE, Ruiz RE, et al. Development of an easy-to-use Spanish health literacy test. Health Serv Res 2006;41:1392–412.
22. Baker DW, Williams MV, Parker RM, et al. Development of a brief test to measure functional health literacy. Patient Educ Couns 1999;38(1):33–42.
23. Wilkinson GS, Robertson GJ. Wide range achievement test 4 professional manual. Lutz (FL): Psychological Assessment Resources; 2006.
24. National Center for Education Statistics. National assessment of adult literacy (NAAL). Washington, DC: US Department of Education Institute of Education Sciences; 2003. Available at: http://nces.ed.gov/naal/. Accessed November 28, 2010.
25. Sudore RL, Schillinger D. Interventions to improve care for patients with limited health literacy. J Clin Outcomes Manag 2009;16(1):20–9.
26. Kripalani S, Weiss BD. Teaching about health literacy and clear communication. J Gen Intern Med 2006;21:888–90.
27. Speros CI. More than words: promoting health literacy in older adults. Online J Issues Nurs 2009;14(3).
28. Parikh NS, Parker RM, Nurss JR, et al. Shame and health literacy: the unspoken connection. Patient Educ Couns 1996;27(1):33–9.
29. Farrell TW, Chandran R, Gramling R. Understanding the role of shame in the clinical assessment of health literacy. Fam Med 2008;40(4):235–6.
30. Anderson JE, Rudd R. Navigating healthcare. Available at: http://www.ncsall.net/index.php?id=1156. Accessed November 11, 2010.
31. Andrus MR, Roth MT. Health literacy: a review. Pharmacotherapy 2002;22(3): 282–302.
32. Davis TC, Crouch MA, Wills G, et al. The gap between patient reading comprehension and the reading level of patient education materials. J Fam Pract 1990;31(5):533–8.
33. Schillinger D, Bindman A, Wang F, et al. Functional health literacy and the quality of physician-patient communication among diabetes patients. Patient Educ Couns 2004;52(3):315–23.
34. Castro CM, Wilson C, Wang F, et al. Babel babble: physician' use of unclarified medical jargon with patients. Am J Health Behav 2007;31(Suppl 1):S85–95.
35. Schwartzberg JC, VanGeest JB, Wang CC, editors. Understanding health literacy: implications for medicine and public health. Chicago: American Medical Association; 2005.

36. Doak CC, Doak LG, Root JH. Teaching patients with low literacy skills. Philadelphia: J.B. Lippincott; 1996.
37. Schillinger D, Piette J, Grumbach K, et al. Closing the loop: physician communication with diabetic patients who have low health literacy. Arch Intern Med 2003; 163(1):83–90.
38. Houts PS, Doak CC, Doak LG, et al. The role of pictures in improving health communication: a review of research on attention, comprehension, recall, and adherence. Patient Educ Couns 2006;61(2):173–90.
39. Houts PS, Witmer JT, Egeth HE, et al. Using pictographs to enhance recall of spoken medical instructions II. Patient Educ Couns 2001;43(3):231–42.
40. Kemp EC, Floyd MR, McCord-Duncan E, et al. Patients prefer the method of "tell back-collaborative inquiry" to assess understanding of medical information. J Am Board Fam Med 2008;21(1):24–30.
41. Wilson-Stronks A, Lee KK, Cordero CL, et al. One size does not fit all: meeting the health care needs of diverse populations. Oakbrook Terrace (IL): The Joint Commission; 2008.
42. Agency for Healthcare Research and Quality. Health literacy universal precautions toolkit, vol. 10-0046-EF. Rockville (MD): Agency for Healthcare Research and Quality; 2010.
43. The Joint Commission. What did the doctor say? Improving health literacy to protect patient safety. Oakbrook Terrace (IL): The Joint Commission; 2007. p. 1–64. Available at: http://www.jointcommission.org/nr/rdonlyres/d5248b2e-e7e6-4121-8874-99c7b4888301/0/improving_health_literacy.pdf. Accessed May 17, 2011.
44. Parker R, Ratzan SC. Health literacy: a second decade of distinction for Americans. J Health Commun 2010;15(Suppl 2):20–33.

Cultural Sensitivity in Patient Health Education

Ann Marie Knoerl, MSN, RN, BC*, Kathleen Walsh Esper, RN, MS, CNE, Susan M. Hasenau, PhD, RN, NNP, CTN-A

KEYWORDS

- Cultural sensitivity • Patient education • Health education
- Social determinants • Patient relationship building

Changing demographics, economy, and political factors affecting health care delivery in a multicultural environment have complicated the clinician's ability to provide comprehensive patient care—especially in providing education to empower patients in their health care decisions. In addition, the new health care reform platforms are reflective of a shift in thinking toward disease prevention and health promotion. To be an effective health care provider and to achieve optimal outcomes, it is imperative that we are cognizant of the social (critical) determinants of health and their influence on individual health of patients. Differences in health can be attributed to socioeconomic, political, cultural, educational, and geographic dimensions.

A comprehensive assessment focusing on these determinants must be completed to facilitate creation of an educational plan that is individualized and tailored to each patient. All of these determinants must be viewed within the culture of the provider and recipients. Today's health care providers are not only caring for a diverse population, but are diverse themselves. Providers are held responsible to give culturally sensitive care. Sensitivity to the valuing of health care technology, treatments, practices, and beliefs by health care providers is important in assessing patient's behaviors in relation to their health care practices. Self awareness of one's beliefs, biases, and personal health practices as a health care provider is essential to the ability to plan culturally sensitive patient care that is individualized to the needs of the patient, with less chance of bias. Often, health care providers assume a superior bias and values that may not be in alignment with the patient's health beliefs and practices. This can cause mistrust, miscommunication, or conflict in the patient–provider relationship.

The authors have nothing to disclose.
Madonna University, The College of Nursing and Health, 36600 Schoolcraft Road, Livonia, MI 48150, USA
* Corresponding author.
E-mail address: aknoerl@madonna.edu

This represents, within itself, an ethnocentric culture in which the beliefs and practices of health care providers are valued above those of the individual patient's. It is, therefore, imperative to thoroughly assess the culture of each patient as well as the culture of the health care provider.

Providing culturally sensitive care during patient education is paramount. The term patient education is normally used to describe a series of planned teaching-learning activities designed for individuals, families, or groups who have an identified alteration in health.[1] *Developing Healthy People 2020*[2] and the recent health care reform platform[3] require us to use a new lens to focus on preventive care. This concept dictates a shift to health education that focuses on health promotion and disease prevention instead of a focus on alterations in health. This upstream preventive approach encompasses assessment and understanding of health behaviors influenced by the health determinants seen through a cultural lens.

Various definitions and expectations abound with the term culture. Culture itself encompasses "beliefs and behaviors that are learned and shared by members of a group."[4] The California Endowment[5] defines cultural competence as the attitudes, knowledge, and skills necessary for providing quality care to diverse populations. This competency is an ongoing process and not an end state. Campinha-Bacote[6] describes five constructs within cultural competence as awareness, knowledge, skills, encounters, and desire. An additional concept that should be incorporated is cultural sensitivity, which is defined as the knowledge that cultural differences as well as similarities exist.[7(p58)]

A second model that is appropriate to apply to patient education and includes cultural sensitivity is ACCESS.[8] This model is practical and "action-centered to facilitate the planning and implementation of culturally congruent care that is sensitive and compassionate in nature."[8(p644)] Application of the ACCESS model offers the health care provider a framework to consciously focus on the cultural factors that influence a patient's health beliefs and behavior, as well as their own, so he or she can implement culturally sensitive care.

Narayanasamy[8] identified six aspects that should be applied to the health care provider–health care recipient encounter:

- Assessment of the cultural norms of the patient's lifestyle, health beliefs, and health practices
- Communication with awareness of the many variations in verbal and nonverbal responses
- Cultural negotiation and compromise that encourages awareness of various characteristics of the patient's culture and awareness of one's own biases
- Establishment of respect for client's cultural beliefs and values; establishment of a caring rapport as the basis of a therapeutic relationship
- Sensitivity of how diverse cultures perceive their care needs and of the various patterns of communications (terms, concepts, tone, and style of communication)
- Safety that enables clients to feel culturally secure and avoids disempowerment of their cultural identity—respecting and nurturing the unique cultural identity of the individuals is necessary.

Attention to these six aspects is essential when planning educational sessions with patients so that a trusting relationship is achieved and to assure that the material presented is relevant within the context of the patient's life view. Success will occur during the educational meetings if the provider's verbal and nonverbal messages convey, "I want to know who you are, what is important to you, and to respect you without judgment." The object is relationship building using the aspects as well as the social determinants in providing a holistic effective teaching plan. Some practical suggestions to consider when creating a relationship and health education plan follow.

ASSESSMENT

Developing any strategy to improve health requires that health professionals evaluate the patient holistically and recognize that the health status of a patient (individual, family, or community) is influenced by a combination of factors. *Developing Healthy People 2010*[2] identifies the determinants of health as individual biology and behavior, physical and social environments, policies and interventions, and access to quality health care. A patient's health status is largely determined by the accessibility, availability, and acceptability of health resources, and directly related to the community in which the patient resides. A thorough assessment and understanding of the patient's environment must include recognition of the impact of educational, economic, geographic, and political influences that influence the accessibility, availability, and acceptability of health resources. *Availability* refers to the existence of services, which are often politically and legislatively funded, and to the existence of sufficient personnel to provide the health services. *Accessibility* means that patients are able to obtain needed services. Services should be affordable, geographically easy to access by public transportation, and offered at times that meet a variety of work and/or family schedules. *Acceptability* assures that services are congruent with the cultural and ethnic values of the patient, including presence of translators and health care workers to address language or cultural needs.

Assessment of the needs of the individual learner should include an assessment of the precursors and factors that contributed to the change in the patient's health status. The health professional needs to ask why a situation occurred before planning any educational intervention plan. Focus on predisposing health characteristics of the patient as well as patient's perceptions and valuing of health actions will aid the health professional in designing an individualized educational plan.

The assessment of the individual learning needs should focus on the patient's

- Emotional readiness to learn—the patient's motivation to learn based on attitudes and beliefs about health-related behaviors
- Experiential readiness to learn—determined by the patient's culture, home environment, and socioeconomic status. Assessment of the patient's ability to learn procedures their belief in themselves that they can learn skills, growth, developmental level, and individual literacy level.[1(p515)] *Developing Healthy People 2010*[2] defines health literacy as "the degree to which individuals have the capacity to obtain, process and understand basic health information and services to make appropriate health decisions."
- Individual learning style—auditory, tactile, or kinesthetic. Teaching strategies should address the individual's growth and developmental level, attention span, health literacy needs, and employ a variety of learner-centered activities (ie, discussion, role play, lecture, group work).

COMMUNICATION

To provide culturally sensitive care that includes teaching, there must be an understanding of verbal and nonverbal messages. Understanding the messages in the context of the patient's culture is essential. Knoerl[9] suggests considering the following strategies to enhance communication with patients that have different cultural backgrounds:

- Be sure to include the family in the process and be respectful of gender role of family members—the extended family may be involved in the decision-making process and key players in helping the patient adapt a new health behavior
- If the client does not speak English, try to obtain a translator of the same gender if possible (preferably not family)
- Ask the patient to tell you about a health behavior you may not be familiar with—by doing so you are honoring the culture
- Ask what the expectations are for the teaching session
- Be aware of the patient's perception of time—if the clinician appears rushed, families may quietly ignore instructions and share less information during the teaching session rather than be disrespectful
- Pay attention to where you sit and how close to the patient you are—in some cultures it is expected that the clinician will sit close to discuss information that is more personal
- Use formal greetings such as Mr and/or Mrs until given permission to be more casual
- Be aware of eye contact—in many cultures direct eye contact is interpreted as a sign of disrespect
- Be sensitive to the level of education and socioeconomic status of the patient—the more education and socioeconomic status the client has, the greater chance the client will assimilate western behaviors.

CULTURAL NEGOTIATION

Cultural negotiation and compromise is an action strategy necessary in providing culturally sensitive care in an ethical manner and in preserving human rights.[10] Cultural groups may have distinct behaviors or beliefs that require recognition and respect. Often, these practices do not oppose the practices of the larger societal group and are easily incorporated into the current health care practice. When the patient's culture is misunderstood, or just ignored, the cultural gap that occurs affects the quality of the health education provided. Acceptance of cultural differences, an openness to understand and learn about those differences, and a willingness to incorporate those practices within the health education plan established with the patient, family, or community is essential in providing culturally sensitive care.

ESTABLISHING RESPECT AND TRUST

Establishing respect for a patient's beliefs and values and developing rapport creates a therapeutic relationship centered on trust. To gain that trust

- Be open, nonjudgmental
- Be aware of the patient's health beliefs, values systems, and how he or she sees the world
- If you are unfamiliar with a health behavior, ask the client to tell you more about it
- Be sensitive to the educational and socioeconomic level of the patient
- Involve the patient in the decision-making process
- Participate in community events and have a presence
- Provide a trusted translator when applicable

- Schedule some appointment times that are reflective of the community in which you serve
- Be aware of community resources within those communities that are credible and culturally appropriate for the patient.

SENSITIVITY

Although this concept is one of the six aspects of the ACCESS model, it should also permeate the whole process of delivering culturally sensitive care in health education. Recognition of the values and practices of those receiving the care and education is paramount to effectiveness of the process. Acceptability of an educational health plan involves recognition of the communication style of the giver as well as the receiver. The above communication suggestions are helpful in negotiating and incorporating this aspect into educational plans. Sensitivity to the cultural influences and context of the client is basic to the success of an educational plan.

SAFETY

Cultural safety is a concept that originally was developed by Maori nurses in New Zealand that focused on individual attitudes and personal cultural mindsets that the nurses bring to their practice that influence how they relate to patients.[11] This concept can be generalized to include all health care workers because it recognizes that "every particular health care interaction is to some extent influenced by the cultural context in which it occurs."[11(p453)] Cultural safety recognizes the potential negative attitudes and stereotyping of patients because of their ethnic background or individual traits. The concept of cultural safety is applied to patient education in an attempt to focus on the underlying biases, professional socialization, and attitudes of health care providers that might influence planning patient-centered care needs. Culturally safe practice fosters the development of individualized educational plans that create useful and positive health care changes for patients.

SUMMARY

To provide culturally sensitive patient education, it is necessary to employ a framework that ensures assessment of the provider's and patient's individual cultural expectations, beliefs, and values. Attention to the assessment of the health determinants and factors influencing educational needs in a culturally sensitive manner is essential for the development of an educational plan acceptable to both the provider and receiver, whether this receiver be a patient, family, or community. Only through ensuring cultural sensitivity can positive outcomes be attained.

REFERENCES

1. Maurer FA, Smith CM. Community/public health nursing practice: health for families and populations. 4th edition. St Louis (MO): Saunders Elsevier; 2009.
2. CDC. Developing healthy people 2020. 2009. Available at: http://healthypeople.gov/HP2020. Accessed November 14, 2010.
3. Fielding J. Secretary's advisory committee on national health promotion and disease prevention objectives for 2020. HealthyPeople. Gov. 2010. Available at: http://healthypeople.gov/2020/about/Advisory/FACA17Minutes.aspx. Accessed May 17, 2011.
4. Galanti G. Caring for patients from different cultures. 4th edition. Philadelphia: PENN; 2008.

5. California Endowment. Principles and recommended standards for cultural competence education of health care professionals. Woodland (CA): Author; 2003.
6. Campinha-Bacote J. The process of cultural competence in the delivery of healthcare services: a model of care. J Transcult Nurs 2002;13:183–7.
7. Perez MA, Luquis RR. Cultural competence in health education and health promotion. San Francisco (CA): Jossey-Bass; 2008.
8. Narayanasamy A. The ACCESS model: a transcultural nursing practice framework. Br J Nurs 2002;11:643–50.
9. Knoerl AM. Cultural considerations and the Hispanic cardiac client. Home Healthc Nurse 2007;25:82–6.
10. Leininger MM, McFarland MR. Culture care diversity and universality: a worldwide nursing theory. 2nd edition. Boston: Jones and Bartlett; 2006.
11. Polaschek NR. Cultural safety: a new concept in nursing people of different ethnicities. J Adv Nurs 1998;27:452–7.

Educating the Patient: Challenges and Opportunities with Current Technology

Jeffry Gordon, PhD

KEYWORDS

- Patient education • Synchronous communication
- Asynchronous communication • Patient portal
- Personal health record

"Patient education is practiced by a process of diagnosis and intervention."[1] Redman further claims that "patient education is a central part of the practice of all health professionals."[2]

Historically if a patient had a question, typically he or she would pose it to a clinician who would answer, occasionally providing photocopied articles for the patient to read. Patients trusted their clinicians, particularly their primary care provider, to give them the appropriate information and education at the time it was most needed.

In today's world, access to information is much more available and no longer has to be filtered through the patient's primary care provider. The Internet now competes with the clinician in providing educational content to the patient. Search engines such as Google and Bing allow the user to type in a few key words and have access to hundreds of Web sites all related to diagnosis. The level and quality of information the patient may access is problematic, as these Web sites are not evaluated or ranked on quality of information and appropriateness for the patient population. Unfortunately the voice of the clinician often gets drowned out in the din of information, both good and bad, that is available online. It is not unusual to see patients confused over what to do, and to gravitate to nontraditional approaches because they have been so advised by friends, family, or even influenced by celebrities who have little or no health care background.

The patient has become a partner, and not just a consumer, in her or his own health care plans and treatment. This situation requires that the patient becomes familiar and educated about all of her or his treatment options.[2] The good news is that there are

School of Nursing, Vanderbilt University, 461 21st Avenue South, Nashville, TN 37240, USA
E-mail address: Jeff.s.gordon@vanderbilt.edu

Nurs Clin N Am 46 (2011) 341–350
doi:10.1016/j.cnur.2011.05.005
0029-6465/11/$ – see front matter © 2011 Elsevier Inc. All rights reserved.

more informational resources written to the level of the health care consumer than ever before. It is relatively easy for patients to educate themselves regarding potential treatment options. The bad news is that there is a plethora of alternative Web sites that appear enticing and accurate. These sites can attract the patient to approaches that are not in the patient's best interests. Educating the patient on how to determine the quality of information has now become a primary responsibility of the health care provider, as the patient is often ill-equipped to easily make these decisions independently. The health care provider's role in informing the patient has now changed. Whereas at one time it was to provide specific information on treatments, now it includes ways to educate the patient as to where to find the best information for specific health care issues and how to make the optimal choices.

THE PROBLEM

The problem is to provide the patient with the correct kind of information that leads him or her to make the best informed decisions possible. The solution consists in educating the patient on what to look for in Web sites, how to commence a search, how to find appropriate Web sites and articles, and how to evaluate the quality of and interpret the information that is garnered from these sites. Then the clinician can take what the patient has gathered, answer any questions, and explain how that information fits into the patient's treatment. In this manner the patient becomes a decision-making partner in her or his overall care, and not just a uninformed consumer of whatever is presented. The patient becomes an active participant in the overall plan of treatment.

THE ELECTRONIC MEDICAL RECORD, THE PATIENT PORTAL, AND WHERE TO START

In 2010 about half of clinicians were already embracing the use of the electronic medical record (EMR), with an additional 29% evaluating the options available.[3] EMR systems consist of a database that stores all of the pertinent information on a particular patient. It can include a patient history, current diagnoses, treatment plans, current vaccinations, clinical notes, and anything else the clinician may find useful and important when treating this patient. Typically the EMR is not considered a teaching tool for the patient because the EMR is not accessible to the patient. However, the data it contains about the patient could certainly inform her or him on past and current issues of concern if it could be made available to the patient. The solution to this problem is the creation of the "patient portal." The patient portal is a filtered, typically read-only, window, accessible by the patient, into the EMR. One example is seen at Vanderbilt University Medical Center. At Vanderbilt the EMR, called Star Panel, has attached to it a patient portal called MyHealthatVanderbilt (MHAV). Through portals like MHAV, patients can access their current and past laboratory results. The laboratory result values, such as a lipid panel, are highlighted for the patient if the results are outside the normal range. The data can be graphed over time to look at patterns and trends before they become major problems. The patient, with clinician assistance, can make changes in diet, exercise, and medication, and observe the results graphed over time. Thus patients become informed about elements of their own health care process and learn what works, first hand. These patient portals also can contain links to vetted Web-based articles, written from the perspective of the patient, for the lay person, making the portal the starting point for access to the most current information related to patients' health care issues.

Some data that are available to patients are difficult to interpret. The solution to this issue is to have the clinical data divided into multiple bins. Examples of data going into bin 1 include lipid panels, basic metabolic panels, and hormone levels, among others. These data are accessible to the patient immediately on being entered into the EMR.

Bin 2 consists of data that require some interpretation by the clinician before being released to the patient. These data are typically held for up to 7 days, giving the clinician time to review the information and discuss it with the patient, before it is displayed in the portal. The delay allows the clinician to view and interpret the data first, before being presented to the patient. It may also allow for a telephone conversation between clinician and patient or, perhaps, even a face-to-face encounter. This approach reduces the anxiety of the patient and reduces the number of calls to the health care provider's office that can occur when a patient misinterprets the complex data they have accessed.

Bin 3 consists of data that never show in the portal record. Such can be information which, because of its seriousness or complexity, needs to be presented to the patient face to face. Otherwise it may be data collected from biological samples sent outside of the institution to a processing laboratory for analysis, which does not have the authority to insert its data into the portal.

A major education component in patient portals is the ability of the system to detect whenever a laboratory result is beyond normal range, and to then so inform the patient that the result needs to be looked at. The patient is presented with a series of pre-reviewed links to Web sites, online articles, or even online videos appropriate for that patient with those specific laboratory results. At one time, this required the development teams of each patient portal to identify and maintain a current list of acceptable Web sites keyed to the patient's ICD-9, diagnostic codes, or laboratory results. It can be a very time-consuming process to track Web sites keyed to more than 14,000 ICD-9 codes. Today that process has been simplified tremendously by the National Institutes of Health, through MedlinePlus Connect,[4] by providing context-sensitive articles based on billing or diagnostic codes. MedlinePlus Connect houses a central repository of National Library of Medicine vetted Web sites, articles, and online teaching materials that can be linked from an ICD or CPT code transmitted from the patient portal's Web site. Anyone developing a patient portal or personal health record (PHR) can take advantage of this free service from the National Library of Medicine.

PERSONAL HEALTH RECORD

The PHR is growing in popularity and can, in fact, double as a patient portal to an EMR. Companies like Google and Microsoft are creating products that serve this purpose.[5,6] The primary difference between a patient portal and a PHR is the bidirectionality of data. The portal typically allows the patient to view only their own data, not contribute to his or her own dataset. The PHR is bidirectional in its data, allowing patients to collect, enter, and store their own data. For example, if the patient monitors his or her own blood pressure daily, the patient can add that data directly to the PHR daily. If the patient uses different pharmacies, that data can be aggregated together in the PHR. The PHR has the ability to tap various databases, including those from a variety of nationally chained pharmacies, and allows the patient and clinician to view the patient's current prescriptions. Links to Web sites in the PHR have been vetted for appropriateness and quality. At present, topics of interest in Google Health have a link to the US National Library of Medicine (through MedlinePlus). Patients can trust that the information they obtain from these resources is appropriate, timely, and scientifically correct. By allowing patients to collect and view their own data, once again patients become partners and not just consumers in their own health care.

Furthermore, the data the patient collects can inform both patient and clinician on the success of the treatment.

WEB SITES

The problem with conducting a search using standard search engines such as Google, Bing, and Yahoo is that the results that are returned are not vetted for accuracy of content, readability, and appropriateness for patients. It is really a "buyer beware, wild west" marketplace out there because anyone can create a Web site and have it inventoried in a search engine.

So how do generic search engines determine content and in which order the user sees it when searching? Search engines such as Google and Bing inventory Web sites based on key words and concepts found within the site. These engines determine a site's ranking by the number of key words inside the site (meta-tags do not count because those are ignored by Google) and by evaluating how many popular reputable sites link to that site. The site gains credibility in the eyes of the search engine if credible sites link to it. The popularity of a site is not really factored into the equation. The actual algorithms used by these search engines to categorize a site are company secrets; this reduces the possibility of a developer determining how to "stuff the ballot box" to raise one's position in the list.

Google does have the ability to record common key words typed into searches. Partnering with the Communicable Disease Center (CDC), Google captures key-word frequency used to search on the word "flu" and has created a product called Flu-Trends, an epidemiologic approach to looking at influenza patterns that predict regional flu outbreaks, about 5 to 7 days faster than the traditional CDC reporting mechanism that was established to encourage health care providers to report on the cases they encounter.[7]

Health on the Net Foundation is a nonprofit, nongovernment organization sponsored by the United Nations, tasked with the responsibility to review health-related Web sites for ethical standards.[8] Sites that have their seal of approval on their page have been reviewed, vetted, and positively recommended by the Foundation. It is an excellent location to commence a search for a health-related topic.

So what are some of the better educational Web sites geared to patients? First on everyone's list must be MedlinePlus from the National Library of Medicine in the National Institutes of Health.[9] The site includes a textbox allowing patients to type in lay terms describing their problem, such as the term "heart attack." It returns a description of the problem and links to tutorials, vetted Web sites, and articles by various professional organizations It may also include links to videos explaining a procedure a patient may have scheduled. MedlinePlus now has a mobile optimized version of its Web site so the patient or family can find whatever they were looking for on their smartphone's web browser while visiting their provider.[10]

If the patient has a question about something in an article they can give the article, or the citation for the article, immediately to the clinician for review. Of course clinicians then need to develop the skill set of accessing an article, quickly scanning it, and often telling patients they will have to review it further. Patients and clinicians need to develop the attitude that delaying an answer is not a bad thing. Rather, it is important to be thoughtful and accurate about a response as opposed to being quick and "questionably" accurate.

MedlinePlus can now provide context-based information, inside the patient portal, directly tied to the ICD-9 codes entered into the EMR. The patient does not have to

search for the articles, as the appropriate links can be automatically displayed inside the portal. The portal programmer can implement such a feature.

A less comprehensive site, but very patient friendly, is Mosby's patient Web site. It covers a variety of topics of patient interest. It is not complete by any means but may provide the specific information the patient is seeking.[11]

Various professional associations and organizations also provide Web sites with links designed to educate the patient. For example, the American Cancer Society provides a wealth of information to make both the patient and the patient's family informed and educated on cancer symptoms, treatments, and issues.[12] The American Academy of Pediatrics provides a site of its own for children and parents dealing with childhood diseases.[13]

Most diseases have patient education materials in a Web site, sponsored by a professional organization. The patient just needs to be educated to first identify the name of a reputable organization dealing with that disease, and then follow it up with a search for the Web site sponsored and posted by that organization.

QUESTIONABLE AND UNPROVEN THERAPIES

Unfortunately, the Web is filled with alternative therapies and potentially dangerous treatment options that have little or no legitimate evidence of success. Unreliable salesmen entice the consumer with slick-looking Web sites, promises of cheap, easy, wildly successful, and nonsurgical cures, and often claim the traditional health care community is "out to get them." Dietary herbs and supplements are the frequent domains of these sites. While some of these products do serve a useful purpose, many are sold without valid scientific evidence or reputable clinical trials to support their efficacy. The National Institutes of Health provides a Web site that looks at alternative medicine approaches,[14] and many disease-specific organizations, such as the American Cancer Society, also report on the efficacy of alternative therapies.[15] Stephen Barnett seeks out "quack" therapies and publishes them on his Web site titled Quackwatch.[16]

Examples of quack medicine identified in these Web sites are claims about the existence and manipulation of Chi/life force (there is no evidence Chi even exists), and that thimerosal in vaccines causes autism in children. There is no current science or clinical evidence supporting either of these two claims, yet Web sites abound on these topics, giving patients all kinds of ineffective or dangerous advice.

PUTTING TOGETHER AN INFORMATION PORTFOLIO

As patients search Web sites, read articles, and view videos, they should begin putting together an electronic portfolio of their findings. A portfolio can consist simply of a file folder on a computer desktop that contains downloads of articles, videos, lists of hyperlinks stored in a Word file, and questions they wish to pose to the clinician (as well as answers when patients receive them). Most of the time videos can be downloaded by installing the appropriate player, such as Real Media, but in the event they cannot be downloaded the link to the video can reside in a Word file. This information portfolio can contain any information the patient finds useful for her or his case. If the patient is concerned about blood pressure (BP), for example, he or she can store BP data daily in an Excel spreadsheet and then plot it over time to look for trends using the graphing tools built into Excel (of course one then needs to be educated on how to use Excel). Some new automated home BP devices even have a USB port to upload the data to a computer automatically. The portfolio allows the patient to look for patterns in the data, organize the material for questions to the clinician, and educate himself or herself regarding diagnosis. The premise behind all of this is that the patient has data and support materials to become informed. Patients are no longer relying on "gut feelings" or the advice of nonprofessionals who may mean well; instead they are relying on real data they are partnering in collecting, and scientifically accurate and appropriate Web materials created by health care professionals to explain and interpret the data and recommended procedures.

COMMUNICATION TOOLS

Central to the education of the patient are communication tools that patients and clinicians can use to ask and answer questions, point patients in different directions, or clear up any misunderstandings. These tools fall into two categories, synchronous and asynchronous environments. Synchronous communication tools require both parties to be online at the same time. The traditional example of a synchronous tool would be a standard telephone call, whereby both the clinician and the patient are holding phone handsets to their ears concurrently. Asynchronous communication does not require both to be online at the same time; rather, a patient can pose a question and check back later for a response. The traditional example of this would be the US Mail.

In today's world we have a variety of communication tools at our disposal. The only requirement for using them is that the clinician and the patient must both be able to use the same tools, particularly if they are planning to use synchronous techniques.

ASYNCHRONOUS TOOLS

E-mail is an excellent example of an asynchronous communication tool. E-mail provides several features, including the facts that nowadays it is fairly ubiquitous, does not require everyone to be on the same e-mail system, and allows the patient and clinician to attach documents that can include text, graphics, photographs, and even full-motion video and audio. At face value e-mail appears to be an excellent asynchronous communication tool for both clinicians and patients; however, there are 4 problems with e-mail that dictate against its use. First, it is not HIPAA (Health Insurance Portability and Accountability Act of 1996) compliant. While some e-mail systems do use a Secure Sockets Layer (SSL) as documented by the presence of HTTPS in place of HTTP in the Web address line in the browser, not all do. Although it is not easy to hack e-mail and hackers typically have more inviting targets, it is not impossible or out of the question either. Second, e-mails can be missed. If the clinician receives hundreds of e-mails a day, one can easily be overlooked. Third, because the e-mail is not included in the clinical record, it makes it difficult to look for patterns in a patient's data. Fourth, it is very easy to forward e-mails on to third parties in violation of privacy laws and policies. Related to this last issue, it becomes easy to mistakenly send an e-mail to someone unintended. For example, what if the person knew two Jeff Gordons with similar addresses? An e-mail could inadvertently go to the wrong one because the sender is confused over two very similar e-mail addresses. So, while e-mail is a popular and easy-to-use ubiquitous environment, it is clearly fraught with problems as an educational and clinical communication tool.

Patient portals and PHR systems are now including messaging capabilities between patient and clinician, inside their systems. Typically a Web site asks the user to type in a message, the user can attach any documents, then the user selects the intended recipient from a pick-list. With such an internal messaging system, the message can become part of the clinical record that aggregates the patient's data in one place, cannot be inadvertently deleted or overlooked (because the system can flag the

recipient until it is looked at), and is difficult to send to an unintended recipient. This system is also far more complex to hack and, if the patient portal is HIPAA compliant, so is the accompanying messaging system that is part of that same patient portal. However, these messaging environments typically have some disadvantages. First, many of these systems do not have the sophisticated tools built into e-mail systems (such as multiple file-attaching and multiple recipient capabilities). Second, both patient and clinician must be trained on how to use these tools and remember how to access them. Third, the patient must remember to access the system for responses. It is separate from e-mail so if the patient never checks it he or she will never see what was received from the clinician. This last problem, however, can be eliminated by having the messaging system also send an e-mail to the recipient informing them that they have a message waiting in the patient portal messaging system. The content of the message is not included in the e-mail, merely a statement that a message for the recipient resides inside the patient portal, waiting to be read.

SYNCHRONOUS COMMUNICATION

There is now a wide variety of excellent synchronous communication tools at the patient's and clinician's disposal. If the clinician actually wishes to see the patient, because he or she wants to look at a skin lesion, for example, or want to observe the patient's nonverbal behavior, video conferencing is an excellent tool. Some video-conferencing systems allow the leader (in this case the clinician) to show his or her computer desktop, which can be very useful if the clinician wants to show the patient a particular Web site or laboratory results, for example. Other video-conferencing systems allow for multiple users to be online at the same time, which can be a useful way of handling support groups involving multiple users in different locations or as a way for patients to get together for common support sessions. Products like Live Meeting,[17] Centra,[18] Collaborate,[19] Connect,[20] and Scopia[21] allow showing of desktops. Skype[22] is currently testing with group video support. ooVoo[23] is a product, like Skype, that allows for group video calls through the Web browser.

There are issues associated with all of these products. First, there is a financial cost associated with some of these products. In some cases the costs can be significant, particularly if they include server hardware, server network connectivity, and software expenses that include client (patient and clinician) user licenses. A low-end video-conferencing system can cost upwards of $30,000 with significant recurring charges. Others, like Skype and ooVoo, offer premium services at a per-user subscription cost, though base services are free. Second, there are personnel costs associated with these products that include training of patients and clinicians and providing technical support to the entire set of users. These products are not trivial to use, and have not yet reached the point whereby they are as simple to use as picking up a phone and dialing. Third, there are end-user hardware costs including a webcam, audio headset with a microphone, a contemporary powerful computer, and a broadband network connection. Then there is the ongoing question of, if a clinician is spending long periods of time in these types of synchronous efforts, how is that time billed? A quick phone call to a patient is one thing; setting up a video conference, getting everything working and then connected is quite another.

Another type of synchronous communication is instant messaging (IM), which typically are text messages that go back and forth in real time. The two most popular generic examples of IM technology are AOL Instant Messenger,[24] also known as AIM, and Yahoo Instant Messenger,[25] also known as YIM. There are several advantages to IM. First, the clinician can work with several patients concurrently in separate

IM windows. There is no equivalent for telephones short of putting a person on hold, which nobody likes. Second, it becomes easy to transmit Web site addresses as clickable links, which reduces Web-address typing errors that prevent the patient from getting to the site. Third, unlike video-conferencing systems, IM is typically completely free. Fourth, these systems work with minimal network connectivity. The only requirements are that both sides need user accounts and both need to have the software installed on their computers. There are, however, several disadvantages to this approach. First, it is impossible to read nonverbal communication because the users cannot actually see each other (although the use of emoticons, which are sets of different types of smiley faces, can allow the transmission of some nonverbal feelings). Second, these systems typically are not HIPAA quality secure so they have the same hacking and security issues that exist for e-mail. Third, the user must go to the trouble to acquire an account and install the software (albeit free). Fourth, it assumes the user is a facile typist.

THREE-DIMENSIONAL FIRST-PERSON SIMULATED WORLDS

Several institutions of higher education are now creating online training in virtual worlds. An example of such a world is Second Life.[26] In these worlds you create a "persona" called an avatar. Through this avatar you can walk, run, and even fly through the virtual (simulated) space. This space can include all of the features you would see in a city, including buildings with public and private meeting rooms, walkways, and even transportation systems. There is no requirement that your avatar even look like you. If you are heavy in reality (first life) you can be thin. If you are thin in reality, you can be muscular. If you are young, you can be older. You can even choose to change your gender.

These worlds are getting very sophisticated, allowing for private meeting spaces where only participants in the meeting can hear each other, while sharing multimedia so that everyone in the room can see and hear it. (These multimedia elements include Powerpoint presentations, Web sites, photographs, video, and audio). Wearing a headset identical to that required for video conferencing allows one to talk (instead of type text) to others in the room. One can actually hear the speaker's voice. Some of these avatars are sophisticated enough to move their mouth while the owner behind it is speaking.

Vanderbilt University is preparing a demonstration-of-concept project that will allow real clinicians to interact with real patients in Second Life. Simulating its Eskind Diabetes Center, diabetic patients will be able to meet their clinicians online in the Second Life virtual world for a maintenance appointment. Data necessary for the appointment will be uploaded into the MyHealthatVanderbilt patient portal before the visit, and although the clinician will not be able to conduct a physical assessment of the patient, he or she will be able to interact and communicate with the patient verbally and show any multimedia information the clinician would want the patient to see. This approach eliminates the need for patients to be absent from long periods of work, eliminates commuting and parking fees, and allows patients to immerse themselves in a realistic environment that holds their attention. Test patients have reported feeling it was very "real." Of course there are some downsides to this technique that will be explored through research. First, the question always arises as to how much added value Second Life actually gives over other synchronous approaches? Second, these systems are not trivial to use and navigate around, so they require a significant investment in training and practice. Third, private spaces in these environments cost real money, which must be paid for. Related to that is who will "build" the virtual buildings and meeting spaces, and how will that be paid for? Fourth, an environment such as Second Life could disappear at any moment, wasting all of the work used to create the virtual space. Fifth, how would the clinician bill for time spent in virtual space? These systems also require a contemporary computer with a powerful graphics card, robust network connection, and an audio headset. The component requirement at the user end is not trivial.

SUMMARY

Educating the patient in today's world is a significantly different practice than it has been in the past. Patients now have access to a lot more material, mostly unvetted, that competes with the clinician in terms of information and advice. Clinicians, their support staff, and systems now have the responsibility to educate the patient on how to find and identify appropriate online articles, Web sites, videos, and educational materials that have been filtered for accuracy, timeliness, and appropriateness for the patient.

The patient portal to the EMR and PHR functionality will become the dominant way in which patients will interact with their clinical record and access their clinical data. The portal will also be the stepping-off link to Web-based materials designed to educate the patient on their health care issues. Products such as context-sensitive MedlinePlus will be built into these systems, making direct access to vetted Web environments an important, if not primary, component in patient education.

Synchronous and asynchronous communication tools will continue to grow in importance and become easier and cheaper to use. As these systems become common, interoperability problems between different systems will disappear, making it easier to use one's own preferred client. Use of video and photographs will become increasingly common. The ability to take a video or picture, either with a digital cam, webcam, or telephone cam, and send it to the clinician will become a common occurrence. Patient-provided data will become part of the clinical record. Virtual worlds will become a component of the synchronous communications mix as they become more powerful in their capability and easier to use.

In short, we will be witnessing a variety of different ways through which patients obtain information and interact with their health care providers, and this will require a re-education of both clinician and patient. Making the patient an informed person through use of a myriad of technologies will become the focus of patient education for years to come.

REFERENCES

1. Redman B. The practice of patient education: a case study approach. 2006. Available at: http://www.us.elsevierhealth.com/product.jsp?isbn=9780323039055&_requestid=602609. Accessed June 10, 2011.
2. Torrey T. The wise patient's guide to being an empowered patient. 2010. Available at: http://patients.about.com/od/empowermentbasics/a/wisepatient.htm. Accessed November 25, 2010.
3. Goldberg C. Survey: electronic medical records pass the halfway mark. 2010. Available at: http://commonhealth.wbur.org/2010/11/electronic-medical-records-halfway/. Accessed November 25, 2010.
4. National Library of Medicine. Overview. 2010. Available at: http://www.nlm.nih.gov/medlineplus/connect/overview.html. Accessed November 25, 2010.
5. Google. Google health beta. 2010. Available at: http://www.google.com/health. Accessed November 30, 2010.

6. Microsoft. HealthVault. 2010. Available at: http://www.healthvault.com. Accessed November 25, 2010.
7. Google. Flu trends. 2009. Available at: http://www.google.org/flutrends/about/how.html. Accessed November 25, 2010.
8. Health on the Net Foundation. Home. 2010. Available at: http://www.hon.ch/. Accessed December 16, 2010.
9. National Library of Medicine. MedlinePlus. 2010. Available at: http://www.nlm.nih.gov/medlineplus/. Accessed November 25, 2010.
10. National Library of Medicine. MedlinePlus mobile. 2010. Available at: http://m.medlineplus.gov/. Accessed November 25, 2010.
11. Mosby. Patient education search results. 2010. Available at: http://www.nursingconsult.com/nursing/patient-education/conditions-treatments/home?filter_id=0&page=1&sort_by=title&sort_order=asc&title=. Accessed June 10, 2011.
12. American Cancer Society. Home. 2010. Available at: http://www.cancer.org/. Accessed November 25, 2010.
13. The American Academy of Pediatrics. Patient education online. 2010. Available at: http://patiented.aap.org/. Accessed November 25, 2010.
14. National Center for Complementary and Alternative Medicine. 2010. Available at: http://nccam.nih.gov/. Accessed November 25, 2010.
15. American Cancer Society. Find support and treatment. 2010. Available at: http://www.cancer.org/Treatment/TreatmentsandSideEffects/ComplementaryandAlternativeMedicine/. Accessed November 25, 2010.
16. Quackwatch. Your guide to quackery, health fraud, and intelligent decisions. 2010. Available at: http://www.quackwatch.org. Accessed November 25, 2010.
17. Office live meeting. 2010. Available at: http://www.microsoft.com/online/office-live-meeting.aspx. Accessed November 25, 2010.
18. Saba. Saba products. 2010. Available at: http://www.saba.com/products/centra/. Accessed November 25, 2010.
19. Adobe. Adobe products. 2010. Available at: http://www.adobe.com/products/adobeconnect.html. Accessed November 25, 2010.
20. Blackboard. Who is blackboard collaborate? 2010. Available at: http://www.blackboard.com/sites/collaborate/index.html. Accessed November 25, 2010.
21. Radvision. SCOPIA desktop video conferencing. 2010. Available at: http://www.radvision.com/Products/Video-Conference-Systems/Desktop-Video-Communications/SCOPIA-Desktop-Video-Conferencing/default.htm. Accessed November 25, 2010.
22. Skype. Skype video calling. 2010. Available at: http://www.skype.com/intl/en-us/features/allfeatures/video-call/. Accessed November 25, 2010.
23. ooVoo. ooVoo home. 2010. Available at: http://www.oovoo.com/. Accessed November 25, 2010.
24. AOL. AIM. 2010. Available at: http://www.aim.com. Accessed November 30, 2010.
25. Yahoo. Yahoo messenger. 2010. Available at: http://messenger.yahoo.com. Accessed November 30, 2010.
26. Linden Labs. Second life. 2010. Available at: http://www.secondlife.com/. Accessed November 25, 2010.

Creating a Tool to Evaluate Patient Performance

Stephen D. Krau, PhD, RN, CNE[a],*,
Cathy A. Maxwell, PhD (c), RN, CCRN[b], Shelley Thibeau, MSN, RNC[c]

KEYWORDS

- Patient education • Education evaluation
- Checklists • Rubrics

Patient education is a critical component of the nurse-patient relationship and an integral part of any hospitalization or clinic visit, so much so that patient education has been identified as a fundamental patient right.[1,2] Patients want to actively participate in their own health care, and to do so effectively, patients must understand their diagnosis, prognosis, and treatment options. In addition, many patients and family members of patients return home with an expectation that information has been sufficiently taught to manage the health care demands of the patient. It is the responsibility of the health care team, and most frequently nurses, to ensure that the appropriate information has been given and that effective patient education has occurred. To determine the extent to which the patient can perform new skills to manage the nuances of treatment at home, a process of evaluation is essential.

One method that ensures some level of consistency in patient education as it relates to performance, and provides a system of documentation that the patient has achieved mastery of the new skill, is a performance evaluation tool. There is little empirical nursing research related to the reliability and validity of evaluation tools, including tools designed to measure patient education outcomes.[3] A comprehensive and appropriate evaluation tool is 1 component of an evaluation process. **Table 1** provides an overview of essential elements that are necessary in any evaluation process. Before a teaching session occurs, the elements described in **Table 1** should be considered to validate that learning has occurred. This strategy makes sure to answer the age-old question, "Can one say teaching has occurred, if there is no

The investigators have nothing to disclose.
[a] Vanderbilt University Medical Center, School of Nursing, 461 21st Avenue South, Nashville, TN 37240, USA
[b] Department of Nursing, Troy State University, Troy, AL 36082, USA
[c] Neonatal Intensive Care Unit (NICU), Ochsner Medical Center, 1514 Jefferson Highway, New Orleans, LA 70121, USA
* Corresponding author.
E-mail address: Steve.krau@vanderbilt.edu

Nurs Clin N Am 46 (2011) 351–365
doi:10.1016/j.cnur.2011.05.009
0029-6465/11/$ – see front matter © 2011 Elsevier Inc. All rights reserved.

Table 1
The rights of patient education evaluation

Right	Questions to Consider	Explanation
The right patient	What is the level of the patient's understanding of what is to be taught? Is the patient ready to be evaluated? What preexisting knowledge does the patient have? What motivates the patient? What are the patient's values related to what has been taught?	Although it might seem obvious, a patient is not their diagnosis. Teaching styles should be geared toward meeting the patient's needs. To evaluate the extent of patient learning, the patient must be ready to be evaluated, care about what has been taught, and perceive meaning about what has been taught for their life. Without these elements, there is no point in evaluating the patient.
The right time	Has the patient been taught what is expected? Has the patient displayed some level of understanding of the content that has been taught? Is it too soon to expect the patient to incorporate what has been taught into their day-to-day existence?	Not everyone learns at the same pace. Some people may have some barriers to learning that are physical, socioeconomic, emotional, or cultural. There needs to be time to identify these potential barriers and address these. Has there been enough time for the patient to assimilate what has been taught to a point that the patient can show skill, discuss concepts, or provide information that forms the basis of the evaluation?
The right tool	What aid or tool is being used to evaluate the patient? Is the tool that is evaluating performance an appropriate tool? Is the tool used to evaluate knowledge an appropriate tool? Does the tool correlate with the learning objectives or outcomes?	The tool that is used for the evaluation must be appropriate and must reflect the learning outcomes or educational objectives. Tools that are incongruent to teaching objectives and outcomes are of limited use in evaluating the extent to which the patient has achieved the objectives or outcomes. Nurses must have knowledge of the types of tools and the level of appraisal inherent in tools.
The right audience	For whom is the evaluation being performed? Is it being performed to satisfy regulatory requirements? Is it being performed to provide evidence for reimbursement? Is it being performed so that other nurses involved in teaching can provide continuity in meeting goals and objectives? Who are the stakeholders in the evaluation data? Who will see the evaluation data and make decisions about the patient?	Frequently, the real audience for whom the evaluation is intended is not the patient. The evaluation process provides internal evidence to interested parties as to the extent the patient has mastered the content, or skills related to what has been taught. Potential audiences include reimbursement agencies requiring documentation that the patient has met the educational goals or outcomes, other nurses involved in the teaching at different levels, or at different times, or regulatory agencies wanting explicit documentation.

evidence of learning?" A thorough evaluation process shows the extent to which learning has occurred. All dimensions of the evaluation process warrant utmost consideration; however, the focus in this article relates primarily to evaluation tools to measure performance.

When asking a patient to complete a task or engage in an activity related to matter that is being taught, the patient is expected to apply their knowledge or skills. Performance-based evaluation tools, or performance evaluation tools, provide the basis for decisions related to the patient's ability to complete a task. The development of a tool that correlates to what the patient has been taught provides a great deal of information when developed correctly. Like most evaluations, performance evaluations can be used for formative decisions, as well as summative decisions. Tools created for performance are an integral part of evaluating overall patient ability to manage a disease process or to promote health. Performance evaluation tools can be time consuming to create, but can ensure some consistency in teaching among different nurses; they provide clear documentation to the extent the patient has mastered the skill and can be safely discharged, or needs to remediate before independent health care management can be certain.

BASIC REQUIREMENTS FOR A QUALITY PERFORMANCE EVALUATION TOOL

Performance evaluations tend to be more diverse than many other forms of evaluation and this makes a thorough discussion of the types difficult. When considering performance evaluations, the range includes a variety of activities to be evaluated, such as oral presentations, musical performance, group or social interactions, and a variety of other activities. With regard to patient education, performance evaluations are more focused on skills that pertain to the patient's ability to engage and master tasks that contribute to managing an illness or maintaining quality of life. Despite the variations in performance evaluations there are some common characteristics that contribute to quality performance evaluation tools. These characteristics are a composite of recommendations by experts in adult learning and education.[4–7]

Any tool that is to be used to evaluate patient performance should include specific behaviors or capabilities that are observable. The nurse is explicit in identifying the specific behaviors or skills they expect the patient to show. Tasks can either be process tasks, in which the steps of a procedure are identified and demonstrated by the patient, or the evaluation can focus on the product. With a product evaluation, the nurse observes the outcome of what the patient has completed, as opposed to the process. Sometimes the product can be the step toward a procedure. For example, one of the steps in performing a dressing change might be identified as "assemble appropriate equipment." The nurse can see the product or the result of this step to see that the supplies that a patient needs to change a dressing have been assembled. A product approach is not appropriate for the full dressing change, because the nurse would want to make sure that the patient follows appropriate aseptic technique in the process. Observing the final product of a dressing does not allow the observer to know unequivocally if the patient can properly perform a dressing change using aseptic technique.

In addition, a performance evaluation tool is appropriate for use to appraise complex capabilities or skills that cannot otherwise be measured with written tests. The performance that is to be evaluated should focus on higher-level psychomotor and thinking skills, specifically application, analysis, and synthesis from Bloom's taxonomy. Lower-level knowledge related to definitions and basic concepts is better evaluated through paper-and-pencil–type testing. For example, a patient could describe on paper how they might administer a subcutaneous injection at home, but this does not evaluate the patient's ability to administer the medication. Knowing how to do something and doing something are different entities. Another example is sterile procedure. One could describe and explain sterile procedure, which is different from performing a task using sterile procedure.

In more simple terms, think about teaching someone to ride a bicycle. The individual being taught may be versed in concepts of balance, motion, and the dynamics that physically occur between these components that are necessary to ride a bicycle. The learner may be an expert on types of bicycles, wind resistance, aerodynamics, and bicycle safety; however, none of these elements shows that the individual can successfully ride a bicycle. Knowing about how to do something, showing the ability to do something, are different domains of learning, and thus require different evaluation strategies and tools.

Tasks that are being evaluated must focus on teachable processes.[8] Focusing on higher-level information, the task that is to be evaluated is one that has been taught to the patient. It is inappropriate to expect a patient to apply knowledge without having been taught foundational principles or knowledge information. The performance evaluation should not require that the patient extend what has been taught, or use inherent insights or intuition, but rather it should require the patient to demonstrate the skills or behaviors as they were taught. This feature is critical in patient education, because the steps the patient is being taught are typically concurrent to a protocol or evidence-based standard of practice that focuses on safety and optimal results of the performance.

Performance evaluations provide information about the patient's strengths and weaknesses in performing a task. The performance evaluation tool provides the teacher with a continuum of information as to the level of understanding by the patient. Identifying strengths and weaknesses in performance allows the nurse to accentuate the strengths and remediate or reinforce information or behaviors that convey weaknesses. The evaluation tool provides a vehicle for immediate feedback to the patient. In addition, an ideal evaluation tool should be simple and concise and should be able to be used by a variety of evaluators in a variety of settings.[9] The nurse should review the tool with the patient before teaching, so that the patient is familiar with the tool and is clear as to what constitutes successful completion of the task.

ASSESSMENT VERSUS EVALUATION

Frequently, the terms evaluation and assessment are used interchangeably, ignoring their inherent differences. In nursing literature, the terms are used synonymously, which is a misnomer to the terms and to the concepts that the terms embody. Persons involved in educational evaluation must have a clear understanding of the distinctions between evaluation and assessment. Although the tools for assessment and evaluation may be the same, the differences between these 2 concepts depend on the purpose of the activity.[10] The purpose of an assessment is to gather data and use those data by interpreting them or summarizing them to determine a direction for action. As it relates to patient education, assessment can be useful in determining what the patient knows and understands before initiating the teaching session. This strategy allows information related to a starting point and provides direction for the education session.

The essential difference between assessment and evaluation lies in the differences in timing and purpose.[11] Assessment occurs at the beginning, and evaluation can occur throughout the education session, as formative evaluation, or at the end of a session as summative evaluation, or both. Formative evaluation occurs at any point once the education session begins. This characteristic allows the nurse educator data related to the patient's mastery of information or skills to that point. Many times formative evaluation provides the basis by which a determination is made to move on to new information or if remediation of what has been taught is warranted. Summative evaluation occurs at the end of the session or group of sessions to determine to what extent the overall outcomes or objectives of the total session or program have been met.

Planning for both assessment and evaluation should occur at the same time. There is an obvious connection between assessment and planning because they both relate to the overall outcomes and objectives. To plan evaluation at the end of the session or group of sessions is often not effective because assessment determines which outcomes are needed and evaluation shows the extent to which the need has been met. How the outcomes are evaluated should be determined as the outcomes are planned. Because the outcomes and objectives should be stated in measurable terms, the method of measurement of both should be considered in the initial planning. Although the same tools might be used to assess and to evaluate, the timing and purpose of these activities embody their inherent differences.

Identifying the educational objectives is the first step in the teaching and thus the evaluation process. Objectives for the skill or the behaviors expected of the patient must be developed before teaching and evaluation begin. Objectives guide the educational process and provide a foundation for the development of a sound and credible evaluation tool.

DEVELOPING AN EVALUATION TOOL TO SCORE PERFORMANCE

One of the most difficult aspects of the evaluation process is designing a reliable and valid scoring instrument. This instrument provides the documentation and empirical evidence as to what extent the patient has mastered the skill or has adequately performed the task related to the management of health care needs. Typically performance evaluation tools are not absolute when actions are unequivocally correct or incorrect. As a result, some form of continuum is usually the best approach to measuring performance. Within that continuum there may be features or steps that are absolute and critical, but these are often accompanied by steps that might not be defined by a certain order or might not impact the overall outcome to the same extent as other steps. This process requires judgment and access to resources for the person developing the tool. A major advantage for the use of a performance evaluation tool is that the score on the instrument and the instrument itself provide documentation related to the patient's mastery. In addition by using a tool, there is an inherent consistent scoring guide, and the potential for subjectivity and bias is greatly reduced.[12]

There are 2 categories of evaluation tool that are most appropriate for evaluation of performance by patients. These tools include checklists and rating scales.[8] Checklists are a list of behaviors, skills, or characteristics that guides the evaluator to determine only 1 of 2 options: either the patient performed the step in an overall skill or did not. However as presented in **Fig. 1**, the checklist may have multiple dimensions, and the same tool can be used over a series of teaching sessions. Checklists are best suited for tasks that involve complex behaviors that can be separated into a series of specific actions or set of skills.[12]

Information received Caregiver _____	Nurse Date/Time/Initials	Knowledge/ Demonstration Good / Fair / Poor	Nurse Date/Time/Initials	Knowledge/ Demonstration Good / Fair / Poor	Nurse Date/Time/Initials	Knowledge/ Demonstration Good / Fair / Poor
States reason for home O2						
States Liter Flow _____ LPM						
Demonstrates correct flow setting on portable tank						
States how to care for humidity bottle and when to change						
States when to change cannula						
States type of O2 system to be used at home: cylinder, concentrator						
Perform changing cannula						
Performs adding extra O2 tubing (use straight connector, tubing no longer than 15 ft)						
States oxygen delivery time by tank and liter flow (see chart)						
Counts and records respirations twice a day. States when to call MD (if count < 20 or greater than baseline) Your infant's baseline RR _____						
States schedule to change O2 tubing						
States when to clean filter on concentrator						
Describes signs of resp distress (retraction, nasal flaring, labored respirations, color changes)						
Outings: Prepares to go bag, and where outings are OK						
Parents perform road trip in hospital						
States safety issues: no open flames within 5 ft of equipment or infant, no appliances that spark, no aerosol sprays, no smoking, secure oxygen tanks at home and in car)						
States safety issues regarding bath time: may tub or sponge bath - clean face with Cetaphil or Lubriderm (no oil based products)						

_____   _____   _____
Nurse Initials / Signature   Nurse Initials / Signature   Nurse Initials / Signature

_____   _____   _____
Nurse Initials / Signature   Nurse Initials / Signature   Nurse Initials / Signature

_____   _____   _____
Nurse Initials / Signature   Nurse Initials / Signature   Nurse Initials / Signature

Fig. 1. Home oxygen checklist used in practice.

Rating scales are appropriate for use when evaluating complex products or processes when the judgment is not based on an absolute presence or absence of the characteristic being evaluated.[12] Rating scales lend themselves to identifying a variant quality to which the patient shows a particular behavior or skill. There are a variety of rating scales, and one of the more useful forms is a rubric.

The word rubric is derived from an ancient word referring to red clay, or writing with red chalk.[13] Clearly, the earlier definitions refer to evaluators writing in red; this is still a common practice among educators in academe. A more modern definition of a rubric is presented by Montgomery,[14(p325)] who identifies a rubric as "an assessment tool that uses clearly defined evaluation criteria and proficiency levels to gauge student achievement of those criteria." Evaluation rubrics have been used in many levels of education to evaluate assignments or tasks, especially essays and presentations. However, the standard outcomes and use of objectives in a rubric are congruent to the development of a tool to measure skills related to health and health care demands.[15]

Rubrics are a type of rating scale that are used specifically for evaluating performance. Rubrics consist of 2 types: holistic or analytical. Holistic rubrics require the evaluator to score the overall process or product as a whole, without judging the parts as separate entities.[6] Conversely an analytical rubric leads the evaluation toward judging the separate, individual parts of the product or performance first, then combines these scores to obtain a total score.[6] Analytical rubrics are excellent for use by experts to identify broad levels of performance and provide criteria for competence and incompetence.[16] Feedback to patient learners is most effective when given quickly after the task completion.[17] There are inherent advantages and disadvantages of both types of rubrics. Deciding the type of rubric that best meets the needs of the patient educational session or program is an essential step in the development of a rubric. An overview of the differences in these 2 types of rubrics is presented in **Table 2**.

Table 2		
Dimensions of analytical and holistic rubrics		
Dimension	**Analytical Rubric**	**Holistic Rubric**
Scoring	Separate parts of the performance are evaluated, then the individual parts are tabulated into a total score	The overall process or product is scored as a whole without regard to separate component parts
Usability	Useful when a focused and clear response is required. Does not focus on the patient's ability to be creative or problem-solve. Useful when there is a more defined process approach and each part of the process warrants evaluation	Useful when errors in some part of the process are acceptable, as long as the overall quality of the performance is high. Useful in situations when performance requires individual creativity, when there is no definitive correct process, only a clear outcome
Degree of measurement	Multidimensional with a total score	One dimensional, with 1 score
Time	Typically involves a longer evaluation process because several dimensions are being evaluated	Usually quicker than an analytical rubric because the evaluator is obtaining a sense of the broader scope of the task or skill
Feedback	More specific feedback is offered because of the multidimensional approach to evaluation. The rubric by design provides extensive feedback without additional writing. Provides ability to give rapid feedback	General nonspecific feedback is offered. Requires additional writing to give more feedback on the skill. Provides ability to give rapid feedback
Communication	Facilitates communication between evaluator and patient	Facilitates communication between evaluator and patient
Impact on teaching	Provides information to help educator refine teaching methods	Provides information to help educator refine teaching methods

DEVELOPMENT OF A HOLISTIC RUBRIC

The steps in creating a holistic rubric are similar to the steps in creating an analytical rubric. Mertler[8] describes a method that combines key steps for the development of both. The first step for both is a review of the objectives as a guide to the task to be completed. This step is followed by identifying specific behaviors that the evaluator wants to see in the patient, as well as those the evaluator would prefer not to see. For each step of the task, or part of the task, characteristics of the attribute that is to be observed are identified as well as levels of performance from excellent to average to less than average. The person or group of persons developing the rubric must visualize what constitutes each level of performance and identify what is the minimal level of performance that is acceptable. In terms of formative and summative evaluation, the level of acceptable performance might vary depending on the type of educational sessions and level of the patient. For example an ongoing class to meet the demands of a newly diagnosed diabetic lends itself to frequent evaluations as the series of teaching sessions ensues. If the teaching session is limited in number and by a time frame, the tool might be used for summative evaluation to determine that the patient is safe to perform the skill without direct supervision. In either case, the same tool may be used; however, the purpose and time of the evaluation vary because of the nature of the teaching session or sessions.

At this point in the development of rubrics, the difference between a holistic and an analytical rubric becomes more evident. The holistic rubric considers the entire task and describes the levels of the continuum that range from excellent to poor, with intermediate levels identified between these 2 levels. At this juncture, for use for patient education, the rubric developer must identify cases and describe situations that show the variant levels. This strategy aids in interrater reliability if more than 1 person is evaluating patient performance. For both types of rubrics, the creator must remain flexible and revise the rubric as necessary but without compromising the quality of the rubric, the rigor of the rubric, and without diluting the importance of safety and accuracy of the task, and the feedback given to the patient. As a formative evaluation tool, the rubric helps guide subsequent teaching sessions. As a summative evaluation tool, the most autonomous and safe level of performance should be the goal. A generic template of a holistic rubric for evaluating patient education performance is presented in **Table 3**.

Table 3	
Template for holistic scoring rubric for patient education evaluation	
Score	**Description**
5	The patient or significant other demonstrates the task in its entirety. All requirements of the task or performance-related objective are observed in the patient's performance.
4	The patient or significant other shows considerable skill in the completion of the task. All essential requirements of the skill are included.
3	The patient or significant other partially demonstrates the task. Most, but not all of the essential requirements are included in the patient's performance.
2	The patient or significant other shows little skill in performance of the task. The objective is not met, because many essential requirements of the task are unmet.
1	The patient or significant other shows no ability to perform the task. No essential requirements are met in the patient's attempt.
0	There is no response from the patient or significant other. The task is not attempted.

DEVELOPMENT OF AN ANALYTICAL RUBRIC

Stevens and Levi[17] provide a framework of stages by which a rubric can be developed to measure performance. These steps are applicable to the development of a rubric to evaluate patient education whether the nurse educator or group is creating a new rubric or revising an existing one. The stages include reflecting, listing, grouping and labeling, and application.

Reflecting

This stage takes into account the educational objectives and overall outcomes. This stage combines the resources and knowledge of a variety of sources to determine exactly the performance expectations. The creators of the rubric consider the purpose of what is being taught, reflecting how the different elements fit into the overall educational scheme. This stage should consider the performance in its broadest context. This stage contributes to the generation of ideas that lead to the development of a high-quality rubric and a clear communication tool for the patient.[17]

Listing

In the listing stage, the rubric creators identify particular details of the task or skill and which objectives are to be measured by these behaviors. Making lists of all of these features helps make sure the details of the rubric are considered. These lists should follow the overall objectives of what is to be taught. The learning goals are listed, and this list is followed by a list of descriptions of the highest level of performance, the acceptable level of performance, and what constitutes performance that requires remediation and additional instruction. Stevens and Levi suggest the use of Post-it notes, because this gives the creator some flexibility to move ideas and concepts and to group in a scheme that makes the most sense and is the closest to representing what is expected of the patient.[17]

Grouping and Labeling

This stage involves putting the similar performance expectations together and creating labels for each group. Some of these groupings are evident. Some have overlaps with other aspects, and may be a part of more than 1 dimension. The groupings provide the basis for classifying expectations into similar skills. For example, it would be necessary to determine if completing a self-glucose level is part of administering sliding scale insulin or a task that warrants its own dimension. The grouping and labeling stage should result in a scheme that has all of the performance expectations related to the learning objectives regrouped into new groups with labels.[17] The objective has a more concrete dimension that provides a more familiar component to the skill, which becomes the dimensions of the rubric. Sometimes a domain might be used as the column label, or the aspect of the skill can be labeled "criteria," or in some cases the objective can be used, and the column might be labeled "objective."

Application

This stage results in the final form of the rubric. The dimensions and descriptions identified in the grouping and labeling stage are applied to a grid format. **Table 4** is a generic template for patient education evaluation using an analytical rubric. The column to the left can be defined by specific criteria, learning objectives, or by domains that relate to the skill. This process varies depending on what is being taught, where, and if the sessions are part of an overall program, or if they are 1-time summative evaluations of skills that are being taught.

Table 4
Generic template for an analytical rubric for evaluating patient performance

Criteria	Poor	Fair	Good[a]	Excellent	Score
Criteria 1 or domain 1 or objective 1	Description that describes the patient's ability reflective of beginning level of task performance	Description that indicates the patient demonstrates performance toward achievement of the task, but still lacking many aspects	Description that indicates that the patient has achieved minimally acceptable level of task performance	Description that the patient has achieved the highest level of performance	
Criteria 2 or domain 2 or objective 2	Description that describes the patient's ability reflective of beginning level of task performance	Description that indicates the patient demonstrates performance toward achievement of the task, but still lacking many aspects	Description that indicates that the patient has achieved minimally acceptable level of task performance	Description that the patient has achieved the highest level of performance	
Criteria 3 or domain 3 or objective 3	Description that describes the patient's ability reflective of beginning level of task performance	Description that indicates the patient demonstrates performance toward achievement of the task, but still lacking many aspects	Description that indicates that the patient has achieved minimally acceptable level of task performance	Description that the patient has achieved the highest level of performance	
Criteria 4 or domain 4 or objective 4	Description that describes the patient's ability reflective of beginning level of task performance	Description that indicates the patient demonstrates performance toward achievement of the task, but still lacking many aspects	Description that indicates that the patient has achieved minimally acceptable level of task performance	Description that the patient has achieved the highest level of performance	

Total score _____

[a] Good constitutes minimal acceptable level; all criteria should meet minimal acceptable level before the patient is considered to have mastered the skill. Requires remediation and assistance with skill if discharged before achieving this level.

The scale labels of criteria, objective, or domain frame the whole experience for the patient, so the labels must be chosen and written carefully.[15] The labels must have meaning for the patient and must be clear. It is a good idea to avoid jargon and be sure that the patient understands all of the terms that are in the criteria column. If the rubric developer prefers to use word descriptors for the row that conveys level of performance, the patient must understand the definition of these words. Often descriptors such as excellent, good, fair, and poor are used, but there are rubrics that use other descriptors, such as gold, silver, bronze, and tin. Regardless of the terms that are used, the terms must have meaning for the patient so that they understand the variant levels and the progression from 1 level to the next.

USING THE ANALYTICAL RUBRIC

When used for formative evaluation the column that is shaded may not be needed. Because formative evaluation occurs during the educational process, which usually consists of multiple sessions, this helps direct educational sessions and teaching after the evaluation. When used as a summative tool for the evaluation of patient education, there is a shaded column that designates the minimal acceptable criteria for evidence that the patient has mastered the task. Although the total score may show that the patient has mastery of the task as a whole, there may be criteria that are not met. In any case, it is the judgment of the evaluator to designate when the level of competence is not safe. In these cases, the follow-up warrants remediation, assistance of a home health care nurse, or education with a family member to provide the task for the patient. To assert that the patient can independently perform the overall task in a summative evaluation, the patient must meet criteria that are safe.

Rubrics also provide a potential solution to the subjectivity/objectivity that exists when evaluating performance.[15] As conveyed in **Table 4**, the rubric can help clarify objectives, criteria, or domains of the performance and facilitate feedback and communication to the patient. The use of objectives also allows evaluation among different health care professionals because each nurse can contribute to the patient's overall mastery of the skill. For example, if the performance is to be the administration of subcutaneous insulin, different nurses work with the patient throughout the day. The rubric helps identify the performance, or aspect of the performance, that has been mastered by the patient or needs reinforcement. Rubrics allow timely feedback, and it is hoped will allow patients to know patterns or problems with their performance.[15]

There are times that a rubric might be a component of a more comprehensive evaluation tool. **Fig. 2** shows a teaching/evaluation tool for patient teaching and evaluation for use when teaching patients to use an incentive spirometer. The tool consists of instructions for the teacher during the teaching session and ends with a section that includes a rubric for evaluating the performance of the patient using the incentive spirometer. Although this tool may look like basic nursing care to which even the newest nurses can relate, it provides clarity, when followed it provides consistency, and it is an effort to make the evaluation of the patient's performance objective. Such a plan provides documentation of a comprehensive strategy that allows for communication among health care members, prevents excessive or duplication of patient teaching topics, and identifies topics that require additional reinforcement and the patient's response to such education.[18]

A

1. Administer Mini-Cog Exam prior to intervention (assess for cognitive impairment).
   Name 3 words and ask patient to repeat (apple, penny, watch).
   Ask patient to remember & administer clock-drawing test (CDT).
   - Ask patient to draw the face of a clock with 12 numbers, an hour hand, and a minute hand.
   Ask patient to name the 3 words again.
   Score Mini-cog (see rubric below)

2. Conduct pain assessment prior to ISTIOA. Administer pain medication if needed.

3. Conduct patient teaching using the following checklist:
   ____ Assemble supplies (incentive spirometer, written instructions, video, DVD player).
   ____ Show 5-minute video demo prior to verbal teaching.
   TEACHING:
   ____ Have patient sit up straight on side of bed or chair
   ____ Support incision with pillow (if applicable)
   ____ Obtain complete seal around incentive spirometer mouthpiece
   ____ Inspire slowly and deeply, raising yellow piston towards the top of the IS device.
   ____ Maintain the coach indicator between blue lines during the full inspiration.
   ____ Hold breath as long as possible.
   ____ Repeat for a total of 10 times.
   ____ Mark highest level of inspiratory volume with slide marker.
   ____ Have patient cough after the 10 breaths with the incentive spirometer.
   ____ Instruct patient to use IS (10 breaths) hourly.

4. Follow up during shift at least three times to assess progress.

5. Complete ISTIOA rubric.

Fig. 2. (*A*) Incentive spirometry teaching intervention for the older adult.

EVALUATION TOOLS AS DOCUMENTATION

Using such a tool to evaluate patient education serves as documentation of the educational sessions and the patient's performance. Thorough documentation as afforded through such tools can promote valuable educational opportunities, resulting in shorter hospitalizations. Documentation of patient education in the form of the evaluation tool provides evidence that patients and families were given information and the patient showed acceptable skill level. The documentation evident in a thorough and well-planned evaluation tool also offers some protection for the health care provider and institution should complications arise and the patient refute that the information was ever taught. In addition, evaluation tools provide documentation of the consistency from the providers involved in the patient's care and education.[19,20]

Even although the Joint Commission on the Accreditation of Health Care Organizations has set standards for patient education and documentation, actual documentation of patient education is under par.[21] The issues related to inadequate documentation are

B

	Domain	0	1	2	3
PATIENT ASSESSMENT & TEACHING	Cognition	Mini-cog: + for cognitive impairment	Remembers 1-2 words; abnormal CDT	Remembers 1-2 words; normal CDT	Remembers 3 words; normal CDT
	Pain Management	No pain assessment performed	Pain assessed during teaching intervention	Pain assessed prior to teaching intervention; patient medicated	Pain assessed prior to intervention; medication not needed
	Teaching	No instruction given	Written instructions given to patient	Verbal instructions given using teaching checklist	Verbal & written instructions given; video demo shown
PATIENT DEMONSTRATION	Mouth Seal	Not observed OR patient unable to obtain seal	Obtains seal for up to 4 breaths	Obtains seal for 5 to 8 breaths	Obtains seal for 9 or 10 breaths
	Coach Indicator	Not observed OR patient unable to maintain coach indicator between blue lines	Patient maintains coach indicator between blue lines for up to 4 times.	Patient maintains coach indicator between blue lines for 5 to 8 times.	Patient maintains coach indicator between blue lines 9 or 10 times.
	Patient Demonstration	Not observed OR patient refuses to use	Patient maintains inspiratory volume at same level throughout shift	Patient able to increase inspiratory volume at least once during shift	Patient able to increase inspiratory volume 2 or more times during shift.
TOTAL:					

Fig. 2. (*B*) Incentive spirometry & the older adult- patient teaching rubric.

numerous, and although with improvements in electronic documentation it seemed that documentation would be improved, it remains inadequate. An evaluation tool would provide documentation of teaching and patient outcomes. It is essential to maintain current and accurate medical records, including documentation of patient education.[20,22]

SUMMARY

The process of patient education evaluation involves gathering information, summarizing the information, interpreting the information, and making a determination as to what extent the educational session or sessions were efficient, effective, and useful.[11] Evaluation of patient performance is grounded in patient knowledge, but is a different dimension along the spectrum. Effective evaluation ensures some degree of safety as the patient shows ability to manage disease processes, risk factors, and overall to improve their quality of life. Although the process of developing a reliable and effective performance evaluation can be arduous, and time consuming, the overall result helps provide consistency in teaching, enhances communication between the patient and the nurse, enhances communication among health care professionals, and provides a mechanism for documenting that patient education has occurred, and to what extent the patient has mastered specific tasks and skills.

REFERENCES

1. Leep-Henderfund AN, Bartleson JD. Patient education in neurology. Neurol Clin 2010;28:517–36.
2. South Australian Health Commission. Your rights and responsibilities: a charter for consumers of the South Australian public health system. Adelaide (Australia): Government of South Australia; 2008. p. 7–8.
3. Watson R, Stimpson A, Topping A, et al. Clinical competence assessment in nursing: a systematic review of the literature. J Adv Nurs 2002;39(5):562–4.
4. Oosterhof A. Developing and using classroom assessments. 4th edition. Upper Saddle River (NJ): Merrill; 2008.
5. Oosterhof A. Classroom applications of educational measurement. 3rd edition. Upper Saddle River (NJ): Prentice Hall; 2000.
6. Nitko AJ. Educational assessment of students. 3rd edition. Upper Saddle River (NJ): Merrill; 2001.
7. Gredler ME. Classroom assessment and learning. New York: Longman; 1999.
8. Mertler CA. Performance based assessments in classroom assessment: a practical guide for educators. Los Angeles (CA): Pyrczak Publishers; 2003. p. 109–42.
9. Wiles LL, Bishop JF. Clinical performance appraisal: renewing graded clinical experience. J Nurs Educ 2001;40(1):37–9.
10. Kirkpatrick JM, DeWitt DA. Strategies for assessing/evaluating learning outcomes. In: Billings DM, Halstead JA, editors. Teaching in nursing: a guide for faculty. 3rd edition. St. Louis (MO): Saunders; 2008. p. 409–29.
11. Worral PS. Evaluation in healthcare evaluation. In: Bastable SS, editor. Nurse as educator: principles of teaching and learning for nursing practice. Sudbury (MA): Jones and Bartlett; 2008. p. 557–92.
12. Tombari M, Borich G. Authentic assessment in the classroom: application and practice. Upper Saddle River (NJ): Merrill; 1999.
13. Available at: http://www.thefreedictionary.com/rubric, Accessed April 26, 2011.
14. Montgomery K. Class room rubrics: systematizing what teachers do naturally (electronic version). The Clearing House 2000;73:324–8.
15. Isaacson JJ, Stacy AS. Rubrics for clinical evaluation: objectifying the subjective experience. Nurse Educ Pract 2009;9:134–40.
16. Nicholson P, Gillis S, Dunning AM. The use of scoring rubrics to determine clinical performance in the operating suite. Nurse Educ Today 2009;29:73–82.
17. Stevens DD, Levi AJ. Introduction to rubrics: an assessment tool to save grading time, convey feedback, and promote student learning. Sterling (VA): Stylus Publishing; 2004.
18. Kanak MF, Tiller M, Shever L, et al. The effects of hospitalization on multiple units. Appl Nurs Res 2008;21(1):15–22.
19. Baker SK. Minimizing litigation risk: documentation strategies in the occupational health setting. AAOHN J 2000;48(2):100–5.
20. Cook L, Castrogiovanni A, David D, et al. Patient education documentation: is it being done? Medsurg Nurs 2008;17(5):306–10.

21. Leisner BA, Wonch DE. How documentation outcomes guide the way: a patient health education electronic medical record experience in a large healthcare network. Qual Manag Health Care 2006;15(3):171–83.
22. Janousek L, Heerman J, Ellers J. Tracking patient education documentation across time and care settings. AMIA Annu Symp Proc 2005;993.

Patient-Driven Education Materials: Low-Literate Adults Increase Understanding of Health Messages and Improve Compliance

Marilyn S. Townsend, PhD, RD

KEYWORDS

- Patient education • Theory • Low-literate/literacy
- Readability • Education materials

The results of the National Adult Literacy Survey showed that about 22% of adults in the United States demonstrated the lowest level of literacy.[1] Another 25% of respondents scored in the next level of literacy described as limited. These percentages represent about 90 million of the 191 million adults in the United States. When considering these data, it is no wonder that often clinicians in low-income communities see a disproportionate percentage of patients with limited literacy skills.

Patient education is an inherent role of nursing professionals. Not only does this include talking and teaching the patient one to one or in a classroom but also, frequently, nursing professionals find themselves in the position of designing patient education materials (PEMs). This task is not often taught in nursing programs nor is it often addressed in continuing education courses; however, most nurses recognize that poorly designed and stated materials can result in misinterpretations by patients. This misinterpretation can lead to inappropriate implementation and/or failure to recall information accurately when needed; in addition, materials written at inappropriate reading levels may lead to patients' ignoring the information provided.

Preparing education materials for patients with low-literacy skills is difficult for the health professional. Many low-literate patients are ashamed of their inability to

The author has no relationship to disclose with a commercial company that has a direct financial interest in the subject matter or materials discussed in the article or with a company making a competing product. The author has no conflicts of interest to report.

Nutrition Department, University of California at Davis, 1 Meyer Hall, Davis, CA 95616-8996, USA

E-mail address: mstownsend@ucdavis.edu

Nurs Clin N Am 46 (2011) 367–378

doi:10.1016/j.cnur.2011.05.011

0029-6465/11/$ – see front matter. Published by Elsevier Inc.

nursing.theclinics.com

read.[1] Consequently, they may avoid admitting their inability to health professionals, making the job of communications more difficult.[2] These patients are often embarrassed when they are not able to successfully complete the necessary instructions. Their embarrassment keeps them from admitting that they do not understand and need further instruction, often using a different format.[2] This issue is a sensitive one and can have a definite impact on the overall quality of the patient education process and, most certainly, patient outcomes that are influenced by patient education.

Some patients may be reading at fourth to sixth grade levels, whereas others may read at college levels. In cases in which materials are produced in English, persons for whom English is a second language may be reading at grades 1 or 2 or lower. Responding to a health survey, written or verbal, poses a difficult cognitive task. Responses to written surveys can be profoundly influenced by question wording, format, context,[3] and visuals. Health surveys and PEMs that limit total words and words of 3 or more syllables and use clear visuals featuring shape and color realism in place of text are more effective in collecting accurate data and communicating with low-literate clients.[4,5] Nurse professionals designing patient materials should consider using vocabulary, phrases, and visuals that are clear and unambiguous, allowing patients to successfully interpret the health content as these health professionals intend.

The purpose of this paper is to explain the theoretical basis and the process itself for improving the ability of PEMs to increase patient understanding of health messages and improve patient compliance. Guidelines are suggested for revising an existing or developing a new PEM for low-literate patients. PEMs should be easy to distribute by a nursing assistant in the clinic, have a favorable readability index, and be easily understood by patients.[6,7] Using visual information processing theories as presented in **Table 1** and methods in recently published works,[8,9] a representative color-illustrated text style for the PEM could facilitate understanding and could result in increased readability compared with the traditional black-and-white text-alone style.

PROCEDURES FOR IMPROVING QUALITY OF PEMs
Developing Patient-Driven PEMs for Low-Literate Clients

Patients are better able to make connections between words and mental images during the learning process if words and corresponding visuals are physically presented.[10] With words alone, patients try to form their own mental images and connect those with words, but this process is more difficult for low-literate learners. Visuals facilitate this process.[4] Getting and sustaining the attention of patients is an element of motivation and a prerequisite for understanding the content of the PEM.[11] Motivational appeal of educational materials for all audiences is important, but especially for those with low-literacy skills. Motivational appeal is an ongoing challenge for nurses as they prepare educational materials.

Researchers who have examined visual information processing have summarized their work as theories; this research has important relevance for patient education. This work can inform the development of PEMs for low-literate audiences with the goal of increasing readability and understanding of the health message and ultimately enhanced motivation to comply.

Applying Visual Information Processing to Development of the PEMs for Low-Literate Patients

Sudman and Bradburn's[12] general principle of formatting emphasizes that the patient's needs must always come first, particularly when the patient's health status

Table 1
Theories of visual information processing applicable to the development of educational materials for enhanced understanding by low-literate patients

Theory	Theory Description	Application to Low-Literate Adult Patients in the Health Care Setting
Sudman & Bradburn's Principle[12]	Priority should be given first to the patient's needs, not to those of the nurse, doctor, or administrator in the health care environment. The medical professionals and staff are not subject to the stresses of the patient	Although targeting low-literate patients, the format of the educational material should give the impression of a professionally designed and printed brochure or information sheet appealing to adults. The effort to improve readability should not result in a product with a childlike appearance. This could be insulting to the adult patient
Realism Theory[14]	Realistic visuals facilitate understanding better than abstract versions of the same visuals	Comparing realistic and nonrealistic versions of instructional materials, realistic materials are more effective in the learning process and, consequently, the preferred choice for low-literate patients being served in low-income community clinics. For example, a photograph of a diabetic patient's insulin monitoring machine is more realistic than a line drawing of the same equipment. Full color is more realistic, ie, easier to identify component of the equipment, than black-and-white version of the same visual
Cue Summation Theory[15]	Color provides more realism to aid the patient's understanding by functioning in a dual role: coding and realism. For the coding function, additional information is provided by the color. Alternately, color can be used to present a realistic version of the visual's content	The addition of visual cues increases the ability of the low-literate patient to store and retrieve visual information. Color in visuals acts as an additional cue to aid the patient's understanding, eg, the white color for a beverage conveys the type as milk without the client having to read the word milk or dairy. Color provides the low-literate patient with more realistic attributes or handles with which to store, understand, and retrieve information. For example, a color photograph of foods to avoid provides realism to the food choices in terms of color and shape of each food compared with a text-only food list. With the inclusion of the color photograph of food to avoid, the patient does not need to understand the text to understand the concept, ie, food choices to avoid
Realism Continuum[17]	Dwyer proposed the visual realism continuum: color photographs provide a more realistic impression of objects than monochrome photographs, monochrome photographs provide a more realistic impression, and monochrome line drawing representations, and monochrome photographs provide a more realistic impression than an abstract visual	Abstract black-and-white line drawings are less effective than realistic black-and-white line drawings for PEMs and health surveys when the realism of color is not an option. Black-and-white photographs are more effective than drawings. Color photographs are more effective for encouraging learning or understanding than monochrome photographs. The more realistic the color photographs, the more effective for patient understanding

is at stake and the patient is expected to implement the instructions in the PEM at home without assistance of the nurse (see **Table 1**; **Table 2**).[12] The patient is under the stresses of the medical procedure and disease management, and those stresses increase when literacy is problematic.[2] The appearance of the PEM has an impact on patient responses, particularly for these low-literate patients. Low-literate patients viewing the PEM should ideally think that they are capable of reading and understanding it and have the impression that it is professionally designed for adults and, therefore, should not be childlike in presentation.[13] The nurse's needs should come second. The needs of the director, health administer, and budget analyst are less important and come last because they sit on the sidelines during the health care process as conveyed in **Table 1**.

Some studies have focused on color realism in instruction by examining visual complexity and information processing. Realism Theory contends that the addition of meaningful visual cues to the text items on the PEM increases the ability of the patient to store and retrieve information.[14] At the same time, the Cue Summation Theory holds that learning increases as the total number of cues increases.[15] Color can function in 2 capacities. First, it can serve as a coding function by providing another dimension of meaning and, therefore clarity, to objects in the visual. For example, the color red for a red apple provides information that the object is more likely to be an apple, not another piece of fruit or round object. Realistic color added to a visual can help explain complex text better than a black-and-white visual. Second, color can be used to present a more realistic version of the visual so that the visual can replace words, reducing the total word count in the sentence (ie, compensatory function). The realistic visual with its color can serve as a substitute for text. Realistic color can help patients understand the meaning of difficult words they might otherwise skip. In addition to increasing the number of cues, color provides the patient with more realistic attributes with which to store information in memory for later retrieval (see **Table 1**).[16]

Berry[16] found that when comparing realistic and nonrealistic color versions of the same instructional materials, the realistic color versions were more effective in the learning process. Later, Berry[14] found that realistic and nonrealistic color materials were superior to monochrome versions for pictorial recognition, comprehension, and memory. In recent work with low-literate food stamp clients, similar results were found (see **Table 1**).[5]

Dwyer's[17] research generated the Visual Realism Continuum theory in which realism cues provide the patient with more information than abstract representations (see **Table 1**). Realism is provided as shape and color. Shape and color realism in a photograph provides the greatest understanding and learning compared with a gray-scale photograph, a black-and-white realistic line drawing, or an abstract visual among a general literate audience[17] and among low-literate food stamp clients.[5]

5-step Process for Improving Existing or Creating New Effective PEMs

Step 1: using existing PEMs in the health setting as a place to begin drafting text

Beginning with a PEM containing the appropriate health/medical content, but targeting a literate audience, is easier and thus preferred. If no appropriate PEMs are easily located, then professionals have to begin from scratch. The text should be revised or developed using suggestions and guidelines found in **Tables 2** and **3** while thinking about the applicable theoretical principles identified in **Table 1**. Complex words such as "consequently" should be replaced when simple words such as "so" are available (see **Table 2**). The former word contains 4 syllables, the latter only 1 (see **Table 2**). "A certain number of" must be replaced with its

Table 2
Examples (n = 22) demonstrating the strategy of replacing complex text with simple words for patients with limited literacy

	Word or Phrase	Letters (n)	Syllables (n)	Words (n)	Word (Better Choice as)	Letters (n)	Syllables (n)	Words (n)
1	In view of the fact that	19	6	6	As	2	1	1
2	A certain number of	16	6	4	Some	4	1	1
3	The majority of	13	6	3	Most	4	1	1
4	Pursuant to	10	4	2	Under	5	1	1
5	Within the framework of	20	6	4	Under	5	1	1
6	Accordingly	11	4	1	So	2	1	1
7	Consequently	12	4	1	So	2	1	1
8	For the purpose of	15	5	4	To	2	1	1
9	In the event of	12	5	1	If	2	1	1
10	If this is not the case	18	6	6	If not	5	2	2
11	If this is the case	15	5	5	If so	4	2	2
12	Concerning	10	3	1	About	2	1	1
13	Regarding	9	3	1	About	2	1	1
14	Relating to	10	4	2	About	2	1	1
15	With reference to	15	4	3	About	5	2	1
16	With regard to	12	4	3	About	5	2	1
17	Carry out an evaluation of	22	10	5	Evaluate	8	4	1
18	Use	7	3	1	Use (verb)	3	1	1
19	The use of	16	7	3	The use of	8	3	3
20	Utility	9	4	1	Use (noun)	3	1	1
21	Modification	12	5	1	Change	6	1	1
22	Conduct a review of	15	6	4	Review	6	2	1

Table 3
Interviewing approaches applicable for use in PEM development by nurse professionals

Name of Approach	Setting	Description	Example
1. Cognitive interview: concurrent think-aloud	1 patient with 1 nurse at a table in quiet setting	Respondent reads sentence and thinks aloud about its meaning. Repeats with next sentence. Interviewer asks probing questions. 4 cognitive interviewing strategies are appropriate here. The first is the think-aloud approach in which patients respond to a section of the PEM and then are asked to describe the meaning of the text using their own words. The second is the use of probing techniques to encourage the respondents to elucidate further their meanings. The third is the paraphrasing technique in which patients are asked to restate the text but using their own words. Last, to avoid potential patient embarrassment, patients are asked to think about other patients at the clinic. How could we make the text and visuals better for these other patients? Would any of the words be difficult for them?	Diabetic patients respond to each sentence in *Diabetes Made Easier* brochure by stating aloud what each sentence means in their own words Nurse notes patient interpretations that are not accurate or consistent with PEM authors Text is revised and retested with same and new patients
2. Cognitive interview: retrospective think-aloud	1 patient with 1 nurse at a table in quiet setting	Respondent reads entire leaflet silently and then thinks aloud about the meaning of each sentence. Interviewer asks probing questions	Diabetic patient reads entire leaflet and then comments on what the content means
3. Unstructured group interview	6–8 patients with 1 interviewer at a table in quiet setting and 1 notetaker/recorder	Unstructured discussion of leaflet with group of patients	—
4. Focus group interview	6–8 patients with 1 interviewer at a table in quiet setting and 1 notetaker/recorder	Structured discussion of leaflet with group of patients. Interviewer asks probing questions	—

4 words with "some" with 1 word (see **Table 2**). Twenty-two examples are provided in **Table 2** for replacing complex text with simple words. Twenty-five suggestions for improving readability of PEMs are presented in **Box 1**. Using 1- and 2-syllable words for low-literate patients is preferred (see **Box 1**). Living room language, that is, conversational style, must be used to enhance understanding of medical terminology, desired health behaviors, and prescription protocols (see **Box 1**).[2] Examples of living room language are shown in **Table 2** (column 6). Avoid medical jargon when possible (see **Box 1**). For example, patients may not understand the medical term hypertension but know what high blood pressure means. Nursing professionals can use their years of experience to estimate patient preferences. Confirmation of those preferences is made in step 3. Active voice must be used (see **Box 1**). "We will ask you about the pills you take" is active voice. "You will be asked about the pills you take" is passive voice.

Step 2: using and preparing visuals
Visuals serve 2 functions. They can explain complex text, helping patients understand the meaning of words they would otherwise skip. In this instance, the visual provides cues to understanding text (ie, cognitive function). In addition, visuals can replace words, reducing the word count per sentence (ie, compensatory function).[5] The cognitive and compensatory functions of these PEMs with their visuals are particularly important for patients whose primary language is not English. When asked about visuals in a qualitative research study of nutrition behavior assessment tools, the low-literate food stamp clients preferred realism in the visuals and the cognitive and compensatory functions of the visuals.[5,6] Applying these principles to PEMs in the health care setting, the end result is improved ease of reading for patients, great understanding, and more likelihood of compliance.

To save time and thus money, the Internet must be searched for appropriate visuals with the corresponding required permissions. Online photo galleries offer the right to use a photograph for 1-time use. The costs are generally $75 to $100. For situations in which photos of patients are taken, the patients should be asked to sign photographic release forms granting the clinic's use of the visuals for educational purposes. Real patients must be used as models who reflect the physician's patient clientele. Physicians should not strive for professional models who tend to be slender, fit, young, and well dressed.

It is the job of the nursing professional to provide health information/educational material in a way understandable to the patient. It is no longer acceptable to hand instructions to the low-literate patient expecting behavior change and protocol compliance to occur and, when it does not, to blame the patient. This process is an enormous challenge when working with low-literate patients. The results of using more visuals and less text in patient-driven educational materials go a long way in developing trust with those patients served. The process described here enhances the ability of nursing professionals to better communicate with patients.

Step 3: testing PEM text and visuals with patients
Cognitive interviewing has been used in the last 15 years to improve the quality of education materials, including health surveys and PEMs.[18] This technique uses theories of cognitive psychology to understand human information processing, including attention span, word recognition, language processing, memory, problem solving, and reasoning. Cognitive interviewing can be useful in the development of a PEM when there is uncertainty about patient understanding of any component of the PEM, including title, main text, or visuals. This technique is particularly useful for

Box 1
Suggestions and strategies (n = 32) for improving quality of PEMs for low-literate adult patients

Using format to improve ease of reading

- Use new header for each key message.
- Use meaningful words in the header to guide patients through the sections of the PEM.
- Use bullets with concise text.
- Maintain the impression that the target audience is adults as you improve ease of reading.
- Aim for a patient-friendly appearance so the PEM looks easy to read.
- Use numerical lists when items need to be understood in sequence.
- Avoid use of italics, all caps, and justified margins.
- Add space between paragraphs or chunks of text.

Revising text to improve ease of reading

- Focus on the must-knows, leaving other information to another venue.
- "Use living room language...language that anyone on the street might use."[2]
- Use 1- and 2- syllable words. Replace words with 3 or more syllables with shorter words or phrases when possible.[a]
- Use an analogy or visual to help explain a complex term that cannot be replaced by simpler phrase.
- Use active voice.
- Avoid medical jargon when possible.
- Meet with patients to get their ideas on how to make PEM better for them. See step 3 and **Table 3** for guidance.
- Use simple sentences of 8 words or less. Avoid compound sentences. Avoid complex sentences.
- Avoid use of abbreviations.
- Use only one main idea in each paragraph.

Adding visuals to improve ease of reading

- Use visuals to replace text.
- Use color to increase realism of photos.
- Use photographs for realism.
- Avoid abstract visuals.
- Color photographs provide more meaning than black-and-white photographs of the same objects.
- Photographs provide more meaning than black-and-white line drawings of the same objects.
- Realistic visual provides more meaning than abstract visual of same object.
- Meet with patients to get their ideas on how to make visuals more meaningful.

Increasing understanding/comprehension to improve ease of reading

- Add visuals using the concepts stated above.
- Add a box to define key medical terms that cannot be replaced with simpler words.
- Provide examples.
- Give testimonials from patients.

Assessing readability

- Use a reading formula such as Flesh-Kincaid or Flesh Readability Index.
- Revise text and visuals until satisfied with readability.

[a] Refer to **Table 2** for 23 examples of replacing 3-, 4-, and 5-syllable words with simpler words.

Table 4
Sample protocol for a series of cognitive interviews using the concurrent think-aloud interview approach

Step-by-Step Procedure	Sample Text
1. Introduction and warm up	Hello Manuel. My name is Samantha Smith. I am a nurse at this clinic. I am the nurse for Dr Fisher. We have met before
2. Purpose of interview	The nurses at our clinic are looking for better ways to provide medical information to patients such as yourself. We think you can help. I would like to ask you some question about this brochure/survey, if you are willing.
3. Time	The interview will take about 20 minutes, 30 minutes at most.
4. Incentive (optional)	If you are willing to participate, you would receive a $10 gift certificate to Target. Would you like to participate?
5. First sentence of PEM or survey item	Here is the first sentence/survey item. It says "…" Please look at it. How would you respond? (Wait) Can you tell me in your own words what that sentence/survey item means to you? Are there any words that might be confusing? (Wait; use probes step 8 if necessary) Can you think of a better way to ask the question/write the sentence so that it would be easier to understand by other patients at our clinic? The response choices listed here are always, usually, sometimes, never… What do they mean to you? Thinking about other patients at this clinic, how could we make this sentence/survey item easier for them to understand?
6. Second sentence of PEM or survey item	Repeat step 5
7. Successive sentences of PEM or survey items	Repeat step 5
8. First visual	Here is the first visual. Can you tell me in your own words what this photo/drawing means to you? Is there any part that might be confusing? Thinking about other patients at this clinic, how could we make this photo better for them? Can you think of a better photo that would be easier to understand by other patients at our clinic?
9. Second visual	Repeat step 8
10. Probes to use whenever additional information is needed	What do you mean by that? Manuel, do you have a word you like better?
11. Preparation for closing	That is my last question for you. Are there any questions you might have for me? Is there anything else you would like to share with me about how to make this brochure better? You have given me excellent suggestions that will be helpful for many patients here at the clinic
12. Closing	Thank you Manuel, for taking this time to help us at the clinic prepare better educational materials for diabetics. Next time you are at the clinic for an appointment, ask to see our new brochure. You will notice that your suggestions are included

patients with limited literacy skills or those from a culture who may interpret text differently from that of creator of the PEM. It allows the nursing professional to examine the PEM's health messages from the perspective of the patient. The nursing professional and the patient may have different backgrounds in terms of culture, experiences, education, income, race/ethnicity, and so forth. Having both the nursing professional and patient interpret the content of the PEM in an identical manner is critical to establishing satisfactory face validity.[6,7,19] The procedure of cognitive interviewing is through semistructured in-depth interviews with a nursing professional such as the PEM author, a patient user of the PEM, and the PEM (**Table 3**). Patient preferences about the overall PEM, including any tables or figures, the title, list of instructions, and general appeal, are valuable and guide changes made in the PEM. A written protocol is prepared ahead. A sample is provided (**Table 4**).

Step 4: continuing interviews, how many to conduct?
The interview process is iterative. In other words, interviews are followed by tool revisions to text and visuals, and then more interviews. This sequence is repeated many times until both patients and nursing staff are satisfied with the final product. This is considered the saturation point.[5,17] This version is now referred to as a client- or patient-driven tool or PEM.[5,13,20] For the final version, decisions about text, that is, the wording, and the content of visuals are made by patients. Decisions about the selection of medical/health content are made by the experts, the nursing professionals. This has been described as the division of responsibility adapted for PEMs, division of responsibility for patient education.[13,20]

Step 5: assessing readability
Assessing readability of the final version of the PEM is important and yields confirmation of success of the cognitive interviewing procedures. Readability is defined as the ease of understanding of the PEM.[21] Two popular readability formulas for English text consider vocabulary, word complexity, sentence length, and writing style: the Flesch-Kincaid Reading and the Flesch Reading Ease.[22] There is no existing method for assessing readability of text with visuals.[5,13] A corresponding formula for Spanish text is the Fernández-Huerta score.[19,23,24] The easiest approach for assessing readability for the English text component of the color-illustrated tool is by using the Microsoft Word software (MS Office for personal computer, Microsoft, Inc., Seattle, WA, USA, 2003).[25] Formula scores are generated for each section of the PEM and for the entire PEM.

SUMMARY

To more accurately communicate health messages, the preferred choice of low-literate patients/clients is a representative color-illustrated text style for educational materials. Using a patient-driven approach identified as the Division of Responsibility for Patient Education for PEM development, these revised educational materials are more patient-friendly and thus facilitate understanding. The result is increased readability compared with the traditional black-and-white text-alone style. Nursing staff may experience less frustration explaining medical follow-up procedures and prescription protocols using the 5-step process for improving PEMs.

This process is an enormous challenge when working with low-literate patients. The results of using more visuals and less text in patient-driven educational materials go a long way in developing trust with those patients served. The process described here enhances the ability of nursing professionals to better communicate with patients.

REFERENCES

1. National Center for Educational Statistics. 2002. Adult literacy in America. Available at: http://nces.ed.gov/pubs93/93275.pdf. Accessed August 26 2009.
2. American Medical Association. Health literacy program video "Health literacy and patient safety: help patients understand" (23 minutes), 2007. Available at: http://www.ama-assn.org/ama/pub/about-ama/ama-foundation/our-programs/public-health/health-literacy-program/health-literacy-video.page. Accessed May 1, 2011.
3. Schwarz N, Oyserman D. Asking questions about behavior: cognition, communication, and questionnaire construction. Am J Eval 2001;22(2):127–60.
4. Levie WH, Lentz R. Effects of text illustrations: a review of research. Educ Comm Techn J 1982;30(4):195–232.
5. Townsend MS, Sylva K, Martin A, et al. Improving readability of an evaluation tool for low-income clients using visual information processing theories. J Nutr Educ Behav 2008;40:181–6.
6. Townsend MS, Sylva K, Martin A, et al. Assessing face validity of photographs to enhance comprehension of the EFNEP food behavior checklist. FNEE Preconference proceedings, Food and Nutrition Extension Educators Division, Society for Nutrition Education. 2005. p. 16.
7. Townsend MS. Evaluating food stamp nutrition education: process for development and validation of evaluation measures. J Nutr Educ Behav 2006;38(1):18–24.
8. Sylva K, MS Townsend, A Martin, et al. 2007. University of California Cooperative Extension Fruit and Vegetable Checklist. University of California, Davis 2007. (English, 7 items reflecting MyPyramid guidelines, 1-page 2-sided sheet for low-literate clients). Available at: http://townsendlab.ucdavis.edu. Accessed October 31, 2009.
9. Banna J, MS Townsend, K Sylva. 2010. University of California Cooperative Extension Lista de habitos alimenticios (food behavior checklist). University of California, Davis. Spanish, 22-items reflecting both MyPyramid & Food Guide Pyramid Guidance Systems and results of face, factorial & convergent validation study; visually enhanced food behavior checklist in 6-page booklet designed for clients with limited literacy skills. Available at: http://townsendlab.ucdavis.edu. Accessed July 5, 2010.
10. Mayer RE. Multimedia aids to problem-solving transfer. Int J Educ Res 1999;31:611–23.
11. Keller JM. Development and use of the ARCS model of instructional design. J Instr Dev 1987;10(3):2–10.
12. Sudman S, Bradburn NM. Asking questions. San Francisco (CA): Jossey-Bass Publishers; 1982.
13. Johns M, Townsend MS. Client-driven tools: improving evaluation for low-literate adults and teens while capturing better outcomes. Forum for family and consumer issues. 2010 15(3). ISSN 15405273. Available at: http://ncsu.edu/ffci/publications/2010/v15-n3-2010-winter/johns-townsend.php. Accessed March 1, 2011.
14. Berry LH. The interaction of color realism and pictorial recall memory. Proceedings of Selected Research Presentations at the Annual Convention of the Association for Educational Communications and Technology. Pennsylvania. 1991.
15. Severin W. Another look at cue summation. AV Commun Rev 1967;15:233–45.

16. Berry LH. An exploratory study of the relative effectiveness of realistic and non-realistic color in visual instructional materials. PhD dissertation, Pennsylvania State University. Diss Abstr Int 1974;35:7717a.
17. Dwyer FM. A guide for improving visualized instruction. The Pennsylvania State University. State College (PA): Learning Services; 1972.
18. Alaimo K, Olson C, Frongillo E. Importance of cognitive testing for survey items: an example from food security questionnaires. J Nutr Educ 1999;31:269–75.
19. Banna J, Vera-Becerra LE, Kaiser LL, et al. Using qualitative methods to improve questionnaires for Spanish speakers: assessing face validity of a food behavior checklist. J Am Diet Assoc 2010;110:80–90.
20. Townsend MS, Hersey J, Dharod J. Evaluation roadmap: measuring our programs and efforts. J Nutr Educ Behav 2007;39(4):S88.
21. Doak CC, Doak LG, Root JH. Teaching patients with low-literacy skills. 2nd edition. Philadelphia: JB Lippincott Company; 1996.
22. Klare GR. Handbook of reading research: readability. New York: Longman; 1984.
23. Fernández-Huerta J. Medidas sencillas de lecturabilidad. Consigna 1959;214: 29–32 [in Spanish].
24. Banna J, Townsend MS. Assessing factorial and convergent validity and reliability of a food behavior checklist for Spanish-speaking participants in USDA nutrition education programs. Public Health Nutr 2011;12. DOI: 10.1017/S1368980010003058.
25. Townsend MS, Kaiser LL, Allen LH, et al. Selecting items for a food behavior checklist for a limited resource audience. J Nutr Educ Behav 2003;35:69–82.

Index

Note: Page numbers of article titles are in **boldface** type.

doi:10.1016/S0029-6465(11)00045-4
                                              nursing.theclinics.com

Moving?

Make sure your subscription moves with you!

To notify us of your new address, find your **Clinics Account Number** (located on your mailing label above your name), and contact customer service at:

Email: journalscustomerservice-usa@elsevier.com

800-654-2452 (subscribers in the U.S. & Canada)
314-447-8871 (subscribers outside of the U.S. & Canada)

Fax number: 314-447-8029

Elsevier Health Sciences Division
Subscription Customer Service
3251 Riverport Lane
Maryland Heights, MO 63043

*To ensure uninterrupted delivery of your subscription, please notify us at least 4 weeks in advance of move.

Printed and bound by CPI Group (UK) Ltd, Croydon, CR0 4YY

03/10/2024

01040445-0011